T0259824

Psychological Medicine

Stephen A. Stansfeld

Noise, noise sensitivity and psychiatric disorder: epidemiological and psychophysiological studies

MONOGRAPH SUPPLEMENT 22

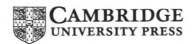

CAMBRIDGE
UNIVERSITY PRESS

CAMBRIDGE UNIVERSITY PRESS
Cambridge, New York, Melbourne, Madrid, Cape Town, Singapore,
São Paulo, Delhi, Dubai, Tokyo, Mexico City

Cambridge University Press
The Edinburgh Building, Cambridge CB2 8RU, UK

Published in the United States of America by Cambridge University Press, New York

www.cambridge.org
Information on this title: www.cambridge.org/9780521439756

First published 1992

A catalogue record for this publication is available from the British Library

ISBN 978-0-521-43975-6 Paperback

CONTENTS

List of Tables

List of Figures

Synopsis   *page* 1

Introduction   3

Review of the literature   3
   Definition of noise   3
   Auditory effects of noise   3

Non-auditory effects of noise on health: subjective indices   4

Non-auditory effects of noise: psychophysiological indices   6

Noise annoyance   6

Noise sensitivity   8

The studies   12

Study 1   13

Method   13
   Sample   13
   Subjects   13
   Questionnaire   13
   Postal survey   13

Results   14
   Stability of noise sensitivity and annoyance measures   14
   Noise sensitivity as a predictor of noise annoyance   14
   Noise sensitivity as a predictor of psychiatric disorder   15

Study 2   16

Method   16
   Noise sensitivity and depressive illness   16
   Experimental design   17
   Selection of study population   17
   Selection criteria   17
   Data collection   17
   Measurement of depression   17
   Symptom Rating Test   18
   Measurement of noise sensitivity   18
   Psychophysiological measurements on depressed patients and control subjects   18
     Selection of subjects   19
     Psychophysiological study procedure   19
     Apparatus   19
     Post-test assessment   20

Results   20
   General characteristics of the patient sample   20
   Exclusion of subjects   20

Follow-up of depressed patients   20
Control subjects   20
Demographic comparison of depressed patients and matched controls   20
Noise annoyance, general annoyance and noise sensitivity   21
Noise sensitivity and hearing impairment   21
Noise sensitivity and depression   22
General annoyance and depression   23
Noise sensitivity and personality   23
Noise sensitivity and recovery from depression   24
Noise sensitivity of depressed patients and control subjects   24
Psychophysiological results   26

Discussion   31

References   41

These studies were undertaken as part of a project on Aircraft Noise and Psychiatric Morbidity sponsored by the Wellcome Trust and directed by Professor Michael Shepherd.

I would like to thank Professor Michael Shepherd for his guidance, support and inspiration. For the psychophysiological experiments I gratefully acknowledge the help of Professor Malcolm Lader, Dr Graham Turpin and Dr Charles Clark, and for stalwart technical support, Jeff Dalton, Terry Hewitt and the Royal National Institute for the Deaf. I would like to thank Professor David Hand, Dr Phil Shine, Linda Jenkins, and Nigel Smeeton for their statistical advice. My thanks for tireless secretarial help to Julia Smith, Brenda Robinson, Dorothy Faulds and Fiona E. Campbell.

I would also like to acknowledge the support of Dr Alex Tarnopolsky, Dr Paul Williams, Dr Andrew Smith, Dr George Stein, Dr Neil Weinstein and Ms Jean Morton Williams of Social and Community Planning Research. My grateful thanks to the many individuals who agreed so willingly to take part in these studies and the consultants from the Maudsley Hospital, Bethlem Royal Hospital, Kings College Hospital and Farnborough Hospital. I would also like to thank Dr John Frank and the Ontario Workers' Compensation Institute for their generous support for my sabbatical during which this monograph was completed.

Finally, and most importantly, this project could not have been completed without the tremendous support, loyalty, and patience of my wife, Dr Jenny Potter.

LIST OF TABLES

1. Spearman correlation coefficients for noise sensitivity and noise annoyance for two three-year periods *page* 14
2. Correlations between annoyance scores in 1980 and 1983 for women with either low or high sensitivity to noise in 1977 14
3. Mean noise annoyance scores for aircraft, traffic and other noise in 1980 and 1983 for low and high noise sensitive women in 1977 14
4. Mean annoyance by aircraft noise in 1980 and 1983 according to aircraft noise exposure and noise sensitivity in 1977 15
5. Noise sensitivity as a predictor of GHQ 'caseness' 15
6. Clinical characteristics of depressed patients in Study 2 20
7. Spearman correlations between noise annoyance, general annoyance and noise sensitivity 21
8. Mean noise annoyance, general annoyance and noise sensitivity scores for depressed patients and control subjects by sex 22
9. Spearman correlation coefficients for noise annoyance, noise sensitivity and general annoyance with PSE neurotic and total symptom scores and Symptom Rating Test scores in depressed patients 22
10. Mean noise annoyance, noise sensitivity and general annoyance scores for PSE CATEGO classes and diagnoses in depressed patients 22
11. Spearman correlation coefficients for noise annoyance, noise sensitivity and general annoyance with Symptom Rating Test scores in control subjects 23
12. Spearman correlation coefficients between noise sensitivity, noise annoyance and Eysenck Personality Questionnaire in depressed patients and control subjects 23
13. Comparison of mean values of noise annoyance and noise sensitivity between first and second occasions of testing in depressed patients 24
14. Mean scores of noise annoyance, noise sensitivity and general annoyance for depressed patients and age- and sex-matched control subjects 25
15. Mean noise annoyance scores and Weinstein noise sensitivity scores for depressed patients and matched controls at Time 1 and Time 2 25

LIST OF FIGURES

1. Noise, sensitivity and psychiatric disorder *page* 12
2. Mean Weinstein noise sensitivity scores for depressed and matched control subjects 26
3. Skin conductance response amplitude by sensitivity, intensity and repetitions 27
4. Tonic heart rate and Weinstein noise sensitivity 28
5. Tonic heart rate for three intensities in noise and tone conditions for noise annoyance groups 29
6. Heart rate difference scores by noise annoyance, intensity and repetitions 30

SYNOPSIS Noise, a prototypical environmental stressor, has clear health effects in causing hearing loss but other health effects are less evident. Noise exposure may lead to minor emotional symptoms but the evidence of elevated levels of aircraft noise leading to psychiatric hospital admissions and psychiatric disorder in the community is contradictory. Despite this there are well documented associations between noise exposure and changes in performance, sleep disturbance and emotional reactions such as annoyance. Moreover, annoyance is associated with both environmental noise level and psychological and physical symptoms, psychiatric disorder and use of health services. It seems likely that existing psychiatric disorder contributes to high levels of annoyance. However, there is also the possibility that tendency to annoyance may be a risk factor for psychiatric morbidity. Although noise level explains a significant proportion of the variance in annoyance, the other major factor, confirmed in many studies, is subjective sensitivity to noise. Noise sensitivity is also related to psychiatric disorder. The evidence for noise sensitivity being a risk factor for psychiatric disorder would be greater if it were a stable personality characteristic, and preceded psychiatric morbidity. The stability of noise sensitivity and whether it is merely secondary to psychiatric disorder or is a risk factor for psychiatric disorder as well as annoyance is examined in two studies in this monograph: a six-year follow-up of a group of highly noise sensitive and low noise sensitive women; and a longitudinal study of depressed patients and matched control subjects examining changes in noise sensitivity with recovery from depression. A further dimension of noise effects concerns the impact of noise on the autonomic nervous system. Most physiological responses to noise habituate rapidly but in some people physiological responses persist. It is not clear whether this sub-sample is also subjectively sensitive to noise and whether failure to habituate to environmental noise may also represent a biological indicator of vulnerability to psychiatric disorder. In these studies noise sensitivity was found to be moderately stable and associated with current psychiatric disorder and a disposition to negative affectivity. Noise sensitivity levels did fall with recovery from depression but still remained high, suggesting an underlying high level of noise sensitivity. Noise sensitivity was related to higher tonic skin conductance and heart rate and greater defence/startle responses during noise exposure in the laboratory.

Noise sensitive people attend more to noises, discriminate more between noises, find noises more threatening and out of their control, and react to, and adapt to noises more slowly than less noise sensitive people. Noise sensitivity through its association with greater perception of environmental threat, its links with negative affectivity and physiological arousal to noise may be an indicator of vulnerability to minor psychiatric disorder.

Address for correspondence: Dr S. A. Stansfeld, Academic Department of Psychiatry, University College and Middlesex School of Medicine, Wolfson Building, Riding House Street, London W1N 8AA.

Introduction

Determining the effect of environmental stressors on health is of current importance because of the increasing pollution of the global environment related to industrialization and population growth. As an environmental stressor, sound has two advantages: it is widespread and it is relatively easy to measure. Sound has some damaging effects on health because of its physical characteristics; for instance, in causing hearing loss. However, the spectrum of ill effects on man is vastly enlarged when noise is considered rather than sound, as noise 'is a concept which by definition incorporates psychosocial as well as physical elements' (Shepherd, 1974). There are two effects of introducing this subjective element: first, it becomes difficult to assess the impact of the physical aspects of sound on man without considering the subjective interpretation of sound implicit in noise. Secondly, assessing *this* subjective element requires self-report measures which are subject to response bias.

Does environmental noise cause psychiatric disorder? Previous studies have been equivocal but have suggested the possibility of certain subgroups of the population who might be vulnerable to the effects of noise (Tarnopolsky & Morton Williams, 1980). The study which preceded the studies reported here confirmed a cross-sectional association between sensitivity to noise and psychiatric disorder (Stansfeld *et al.* 1985*a*, *b*). Sensitivity to noise is a measure of attitudes to noise in general which also predicts annoyance reactions to noise. Because of the association of noise sensitivity and psychiatric disorder, the question may be asked, is noise sensitivity an indicator of this vulnerable subgroup who are at high risk for psychiatric disorder?

This monograph investigates the proposition that the subjective interpretation of sound as noise, and by those who are sensitive to noise, is central to the mechanism of the ill effects of noise on man in relation to psychiatric disorder using both subjective and psychophysiological methods. Psychophysiological measurements are used both to complement and provide external validation for the subjective measurements.

REVIEW OF THE LITERATURE

This literature review examines the evidence for the effects of noise on man with particular reference to individual differences in effects on health. Further details of these health effects may be found elsewhere (Kryter, 1970, 1985; McLean & Tarnopolsky, 1977; Tarnopolsky & Clark, 1984; Loeb, 1986; Stansfeld, 1989).

Definition of noise

Noise is often defined as 'unwanted sound', perceived as harmful or unpleasant. It might seem tautologous to argue whether noise harms health. It is not necessarily so because the perception of the unpleasantness of noise is not synonymous with measurable ill effects on health. To an extent 'one person's music is another person's noise' but in practice, there is a common western consensus that sound from factory machinery, aircraft, road vehicles and trains is noisome (Cameron *et al.* 1972) and constitutes a source of environmental pollution. In one area of enquiry there is good evidence that noise harms health, i.e. hearing loss related to the objective physical properties of the sound rather than its subjective interpretation. It is a natural starting point in reviewing the ill effects of noise on health.

Auditory effects of noise

Sound, manifest as environmental noise, has temporary or permanent effects of noise-induced hearing loss (Burns, 1973). Exposure to higher intensity and certain types of noise may increase this risk but there is also evidence of individual susceptibility (Kryter, 1985). Psychological disorder may arise secondary to the difficulty in communication, and hence social isolation resulting from hearing loss, with greater psychological disorder in those with bilateral as opposed to unilateral hearing loss (Mahapatra, 1974), or both psychological disorder and hearing loss may arise from shared social origins. Severe mental illness is often paranoid rather than depressive in nature in those with hearing loss (Kay & Roth, 1961; Cooper *et al.* 1974).

NON-AUDITORY EFFECTS OF NOISE ON HEALTH: SUBJECTIVE INDICES

Noise exposure and symptoms

Apart from the auditory effects of noise on health there is little convincing evidence that noise causes physical illness. Evidence of the effect of noise on the cardiovascular system is equivocal (Thompson, 1983, 1991; Babisch et al. 1988; Ising et al. 1990); the balance is in favour of noise raising blood pressure, with the most striking effects in school children exposed to aircraft noise (Cohen et al. 1980; Cohen & Weinstein, 1981) and those already hypertensive (Arguelles et al. 1970).

Symptoms among industrial workers regularly exposed to high noise levels in settings such as weaving mills (Granati et al. 1959), jet aircraft test beds (Bugard et al. 1953), schools near Heathrow Airport (Crook & Langdon, 1974) and factories (Melamed et al. 1988) include nausea, headaches, argumentativeness, changes in mood, anxiety and sexual impotence. More self-reported illness and illness-related absenteeism (Cameron et al. 1972), social conflicts at work and home (Jansen, 1961) and actual absenteeism (Cohen, 1976) has also been found in noisy rather than quiet industries. Many of these industrial studies are difficult to interpret because workers were exposed to other stressors in addition to excess noise, such as physical danger and heavy work demands, which may be far more potent than noise in causing symptoms. There may also be differential selection of individuals working in noisy areas. For instance, jobs in noisy areas may be less desirable, may be more difficult to fill, and hence may attract individuals with health problems which have prevented them from attaining more desirable jobs. On the other hand, jobs in high noise-exposure areas may be dangerous and demand toughness and resilience not required for jobs in quieter areas. This applies to a study of men working on aircraft carriers (Davis, 1958), which revealed very few symptoms among those men exposed to high noise levels. It seems likely that these men were a very highly selected group from whom those who might have been expected to react adversely to noise had been excluded.

Environmental noise, though less intense, tends to be more difficult for the ordinary citizen to avoid. Community surveys have found that high percentages of people reported 'headaches', 'restless nights' and 'being tense and edgy' in high noise areas around Heathrow (OPCS, 1971), and similarly around Osaka airport in Japan (Kokokushka, 1973) and Germany (Finke et al. 1974), and for traffic noise in Sweden (Öhrström, 1989). An explicit link between aircraft noise and symptoms in these studies raises the possibility of bias towards over-reporting of symptoms in those wishing to influence the results of the study (Barker & Tarnopolsky, 1978). It is notable that Grandjean's study around three Swiss airports (Grandjean et al. 1973), which did not mention that the study was related to aircraft noise, did not find an association between aircraft noise exposure level and symptoms. In the West London Survey (Tarnopolsky et al. 1980) 'tinnitus', 'burns, cuts and minor accidents', 'ear problems' and 'skin troubles' were more common in high aircraft noise exposure areas. Acute symptoms were more common in high noise, in particular, 'depression', 'irritability', 'difficulty getting off to sleep', 'night waking', 'skin troubles', 'swollen ankles', and 'burns, cuts and minor accidents'. However, apart from 'ear problems' and 'tinnitus', 20 out of 23 chronic symptoms were more common in low noise. Symptoms did not increase with increasing levels of noise. This is possibly related to more social disadvantage and associated ill-health among residents in low aircraft noise exposure areas and the unwillingness of chronically unhealthy individuals to move into potentially stressful high noise exposure areas. Nevertheless, this does not exclude an effect of noise in causing some acute psychological symptoms and it may be that many of the effects of noise in industrial and teaching settings relate to disturbances in communication. If noise may lead to some psychological symptoms, does noise exposure go on to cause psychiatric disorder? The evidence relating noise to psychiatric ill-health is described below.

Noise exposure and mental hospital admission rates

Much of the concern with the possible effects of noise on mental health began with the study of admissions to psychiatric hospitals from noisy areas. Early studies (Abey-Wickrama et al. 1969; Meecham & Smith, 1977; Meecham & Shaw, 1979) found associations between aircraft noise level and mental hospital admissions in London and Los Angeles. These have been criticized on methodological grounds (Chowns, 1970; Frerichs *et al.* 1980) and a replication study of Abey-Wickrama's study in London, by Gattoni & Tarnopolsky (1973) failed to confirm these findings. Jenkins *et al.* (1979) found age standardized admission rates to Springfield Hospital over four years were higher as the level of noise decreased, but lower noise areas were also central urban districts where high admission rates would be expected. In a further study (Jenkins *et al.* 1981), 9000 admissions to three psychiatric hospitals (1969–72) over a four-year period were compared: Springfield Hospital, St Bernard's Hospital and Holloway Sanatorium. In the latter two hospitals high aircraft noise was associated with higher admission rates, but in all three hospitals the trends of admission rates seemed to follow more closely non-noise factors and the effect of noise, if any, could only be moderating the effect of other causal variables but not overriding them.

Kryter (1985, 1990) criticizes Jenkins *et al.* (1981) and in a re-analysis of the data found 'a more consistently positive relation between level of exposure to aircraft noise and admission rates...' Suffice it to say the route to hospitalization is influenced by many psychosocial variables more potent than noise exposure and whether noise causes mental illness is more suitably answered by studying a community sample.

Noise exposure and psychiatric morbidity in the community

In a pilot study carried out in the community in West London using high aircraft noise areas around Heathrow airport Tarnopolsky *et al.* (1978) found no association between noise exposure and either General Health Questionnaire (GHQ) scores (Goldberg, 1972), (dichotomized 4/5, low scorers/high scorers) or estimated psychiatric cases (Goldberg *et al.* 1970); even when road traffic noise exposure was controlled. There were differences in prevalence of psychiatric morbidity according to noise exposure in three subgroups; persons 'aged 15–44 of high education' (41%, 14% $P < 0.05$), 'women aged 15–44' (30%, 13% NS) and those in 'professional or managerial occupations'. In a subsequent log-linear analysis they found

that the combination of education and noise together had a substantial effect on the GHQ score and expressed the guarded opinion that noise might have an effect in causing morbidity within certain vulnerable subgroups.

In the subsequent West London Survey of Psychiatric Morbidity (Tarnopolsky & Morton Williams, 1980), 5885 adults were randomly selected, stratified within four aircraft noise zones (< 35NNI, 35–44NNI, 45–54NNI, > 55NNI) according to the Noise and Number Index (NNI). In this study, as in the pilot study, no overall relationship was found between aircraft noise and the prevalence of psychiatric morbidity either for GHQ scores or for estimated psychiatric cases, using various indices of noise exposure. There was an association between noise and psychiatric morbidity in two subgroups: 'finished full time education at aged > 19 years', and 'professionals'. These two categories which showed a strong association were combined and did show a significant association between noise and psychiatric morbidity ($\chi^2 = 8.18$, df 3 $P < 0.05$). However, this association became statistically insignificant when estimated cases rather than GHQ scores were used. Tarnopolsky & Morton Williams (1980) conclude 'our results show so far that noise *per se* in the community at large, does not seem to be a frequent, severe, pathogenic factor in causing mental *illness* but that it is associated with symptomatic response in selected subgroups of the population'.

Health services use by noise exposure has also been used to observe the relationship between noise and psychiatric disorder. Grandjean *et al.* (1973) reported that the proportion of the population taking drugs was higher in areas with high levels of aircraft noise and Knipshild & Oudshoorn (1977) found the purchase of sleeping pills, antacids, sedative and antihypertensive drugs all increased in a village newly exposed to noise, but not in a 'control' village where the noise level remained unchanged. Both these investigations also found an association between general practitioner contact rate and level of noise exposure. In the Heathrow study (Watkins *et al.* 1981) various health-care indicators were used, namely the use of any drug, any specifically psychiatric or self-prescribed drugs in the last two weeks, as well as visits to the general practitioner, attendance at out-patients or in-patients in the last three months, and the use of various community and health services. There was no clear trend for any of these indicators in relation to noise.

Effects of noise on performance

These negative findings are, in many ways, surprising for there is good evidence that noise has significant effects on performance (Loeb, 1986) and sleep and in causing annoyance and it might be expected that these disturbances might be expressed as psychiatric disorder.

The general themes of the many complex noise influences on performance are that noise increases arousal, and decreases attention through distraction (Broadbent, 1953), increased focusing or attention to irrelevant stimuli (Cohen & Spacapan, 1978), and latterly that noise alters choice of task strategy (Smith & Broadbent, 1981). Even relatively low levels of noise may have subtle ill-effects and the state of the person at the time of performance may be as important as the noise itself (Broadbent, 1983). There are some individual differences in performance decrements related to neuroticism and extraversion (Von Wright & Vauras, 1980) and performance decrements are increased under multiple task conditions (Hockey, 1970). Noise may also affect social performance as: (1) a stressor causing unwanted aversive changes in affective state; (2) by masking speech and impairing communication; and (3) by distracting attention from relevant social cues (Jones et al. 1981). It may be that people whose performance strategies are already limited for other reasons (e.g. high anxiety), and who are faced with multiple tasks may be more vulnerable to the masking and distracting effects of noise.

Effects of noise on sleep

There is both objective and subjective evidence for sleep disturbance by noise (Öhrström, 1982; Öhrström et al. 1988a). Moreover, there are repeated findings of individual differences in susceptibility to sleep disturbance which include noise awakenings from sonic booms in soldiers scoring highly on neuroticism (Rylander et al. 1972), worse sleep quality, more awakenings and more morning tiredness in noise sensitive students (Öhrström & Bjorkman, 1988) and more reported sleep disturbance in noise sensitive people from community surveys (Civil Aviation

Authority, 1980). Noise effects on sleep may habituate over time (Vallet & Francois, 1982) but small sleep deficits may persist for years (Globus et al. 1973).

NON-AUDITORY EFFECTS OF NOISE: PSYCHOPHYSIOLOGICAL INDICES

If noise has these effects on performance and sleep, what is the underlying response of the autonomic nervous system to noise? The immediate, autonomically mediated physiological response to noise exposure is the orientating reflex which rapidly habituates unless the stimulus is novel, indicates conflict, or has learned significance (Sokolov, 1963; Lynn, 1966). A small number of people do not habituate (Jansen, 1969) and it may be that this group perceive a chronic threat from noise. It is not clear either whether this group with chronic arousal will develop long-term ill effects on health or whether they perceive such a vulnerability. Certainly, the meaning of the noise is important in determining physiological effects, as noise induced vasoconstriction was found to persist longer under conditions of perceived uncontrollability (Glass & Singer, 1972). Considering other physiological indicators: noise induces inconsistent effects on the endocrine system, usually increasing secretion of adrenal medullary and cortical hormones in short-term responses, but possible long-term effects have been little studied (Arguelles, 1967; Atherley et al. 1970; Beardwood, 1982).

NOISE ANNOYANCE

Overall, there are persistent physiological reactions to noise in a minority who find noise threatening. There are performance and sleep decrements in noise which are partially related (a) to the meaning of the noise, and (b) to personality characteristics such as neuroticism and extraversion. However, the most widespread and well-documented subjective response to noise is annoyance. Cohen & Weinstein, (1981) state 'in some cases annoyance may be fear or simply aversiveness, but many of the correlates of annoyance are predictable if one views annoyance as a mild form of anger...produced when people believe that they have been harmed and that the harm was both avoidable and undeserved'. Wilson (1963) further emphasized the intrusiveness of noise into personal privacy and that the meaning of a noise, for any individual, is important in determining whether that individual will be annoyed by it (Gunn, 1987). Annoyance reactions to noise are often associated with reported interference of noise in everyday activities. This interference probably precedes and leads on to annoyance (Taylor, 1984; Hall *et al.* 1985). Annoyance is also dependent on the context in which the noise is heard. Overall, it seems that conversation and watching television or listening to the radio (all involving speech communication) are the activities most disturbed by aircraft noise (Hall *et al.* 1985) while traffic noise, if present at night, is most disturbing for sleep. Disturbances of communication may be particularly important in the development of psychiatric disorders, as seen in the association between deafness and psychiatric disorder.

Noise annoyance, noise and symptoms

In the studies on noise and psychiatric disorder it became clear that it was easier to interpret the results if noise annoyance was also considered. For noise annoyance is associated, not only with noise level, but also with expression of symptoms and formal psychiatric disorder. In the West London Survey, respondents exhibiting more noise annoyance also displayed the most symptoms, both acute and chronic, in both high and low noise exposure areas confirming earlier studies (Fog & Jonsson, 1968). A question arises from this, if there is a strong link between noise and annoyance, and those who are highly annoyed showed the greatest number of symptoms then why are symptoms not more common in the high noise area? This apparent paradox might be explained by the 'Vulnerability Hypothesis' (Tarnopolsky *et al.* 1980). According to this explanation, noise is not directly pathogenic but sorts individuals into annoyance categories according to their vulnerability to stress. Thus, at any noise level there may be some individuals who take little notice of the noise and some who are extremely annoyed by it. In *low noise* conditions, a high annoyance response indicates a high degree of vulnerability, while those who display little annoyance are more representative of the population. In *high noise* conditions those who display little an-

noyance are assumed to be least vulnerable, while those expressing high annoyance would include both vulnerable individuals and those representative of the general population disturbed by noise. The pattern of symptoms does fit this hypothesis (Tarnopolsky *et al.* 1980).

Noise exposure, annoyance and psychiatric morbidity

Tarnopolsky *et al.* (1978) found that noise and GHQ scores were the strongest predictors of annoyance and that a high GHQ score led to annoyance rather than high annoyance leading to psychiatric morbidity. Tarnopolsky & Morton Williams (1980) found that a high GHQ score intensified the expression of annoyance, regardless of the level of noise exposure, but did not modify substantially the distribution of annoyance in relation to noise. They conclude 'therefore when the level of noise is not sufficient to justify the extreme annoyance, it is those people with a psychiatric disturbance who are likely to be intensely annoyed and who constitute about two-thirds of the small proportion who are very annoyed there'. They say that there is little evidence to suggest that annoyance acts as an intervening variable between noise and morbidity. Here, as Kasl points out (1984), is the intriguing situation of an intervening variable which does not intervene. However, it may be that there are two processes at work here.

Noise and non-noise predictors of the annoyance response

What are the other predictors of noise annoyance? Although psychiatric disorder predicts noise annoyance, noise level and other non-acoustic factors[1] are more strongly related to

[1] Among factors predicting annoyance, acoustic factors include loudness (Berglund *et al.* 1976), duration (McKennell, 1977), frequency and impulsiveness of noise (Job, 1988), and the presence of accompanying vibration with the complex interactions with background noise and the number of noise events (Langdon, 1976*a*; Stephens & Powell, 1978; Fields, 1984). Non-acoustic factors predicting annoyance include demographic factors, fear of the noise or noise source (Gunn *et al.* 1981; Moran *et al.* 1981; Bullen *et al.* 1986) and attitudes to the noise source (TRACOR, 1971; Borsky, 1980). These include the predictability and controllability of the noise (Graeven, 1975), general dislike of the environment (McKennell, 1963; Langdon, 1976*b*) and attitudes to the noise source including misfeasance (Borsky, 1961, Hazard, 1971; Rylander *et al.* 1972; Finke, 1974, Jonah *et al.* 1981). There is some limited evidence that personality traits, such as extraversion (Shigehisa & Gunn, 1979; Ohrström *et al.* 1988*b*) predict annoyance and relate to better performance in noise (Gulian, 1974, Davies & Hockey, 1966), although some studies have found negative results (Griffiths & Delauzun, 1977; Raw & Griffiths, 1988).

noise annoyance. Noise level is associated with annoyance in a dose-response relationship in both traffic and aircraft noise studies (McKennell, 1963; Griffiths & Langdon, 1968; Schultz, 1978; Tarnopolsky & Morton Williams, 1980). While average population measures of noise annoyance (either mean or median) agree fairly strongly with noise exposure (mean $r = 0.82$); Job, 1988), the association between individuals' annoyance responses and noise exposure is very much smaller (mean $r = 0.42$; Job, 1988; Griffiths & Langdon, 1968; Langdon, 1976b; Schultz, 1978; Vallet et al. 1978; Jonah et al. 1981). That is to say, at any particular noise exposure level there is a wide individual variation in the degree of annoyance felt or expressed. Individual variance in annoyance can be explained in terms of differences in noise exposure estimation, errors in measurement of annoyance, the context of the response, adaptation to noise, population sampling problems and individual differences (Evans & Tafalla, 1987; Langdon 1987; Job, 1988). Differences in noise exposure estimation between individuals can be important but Job (1988) has pointed out that individual factors such as noise sensitivity and attitudes to noise sources account for more variance than noise exposure.

NOISE SENSITIVITY

Two separate but related concepts of noise sensitivity can be identified (McKennell, 1963). First, there is *sensitivity to annoyance* by noise which identifies individuals as being highly sensitive when they express more annoyance than their neighbours for a particular level of noise (Griffiths & Langdon, 1968; Bregman & Pearson, 1972) and being low sensitive or 'imperturbable' when they express lower levels of annoyance than their neighbours. Secondly, *general susceptibility to noise*, which is associated with annoyance, but implies susceptibility to a wide range of noises. Anderson's (1971) definition distinguishes sensitivity from annoyance: "it should be possible to disentangle one factor involving underlying attitudes towards noise in general (i.e. sensitivity) as well as another, concerning attitudes towards a specified noise or noise environment (i.e. annoyance)'. The operational definition of noise sensitivity used in this monograph is Anderson's (1971): noise

sensitivity measures attitudes to noise in general.

In community surveys noise sensitivity has usually been measured by short direct questions asking about noise sensitivity, or lists of annoying noises (Bennett, 1945; Langdon, 1976b; Griffiths & Delauzun, 1977; Tarnopolsky & Morton-Williams, 1980; Bullen et al. 1986; Raw & Griffiths, 1988). In laboratory studies larger questionnaires have been used (Bowsher et al. 1966; Anderson, 1971; Broadbent, 1972; Bregman & Pearson, 1972; Weinstein, 1978). The internal reliability of measures is fairly high ($r = 0.76$–0.88) while repeatability is less consistent ($r = 0.35$–0.75) depending on type and sophistication of the measures. Tarnopolsky & Morton Williams (1980) report that 19% of the population say that they are more sensitive to noise than average. Few demographic factors seem to relate to noise sensitivity although many samples, studied in the laboratory, have not been representative of the population (Anderson, 1971; Moreira & Bryan, 1972). Noise sensitivity does not differ by sex (Langdon, 1976c) but has generally been found to increase with age (Jonsson, 1964; Broadbent, 1972; Langdon, 1976c; Ising et al. 1980; Thomas & Jones, 1982), particularly in women. Where it has been reviewed middle-class subjects have sometimes been found to be marginally more sensitive to noise (OPCS, 1971; Meijer et al. 1985).

Noise sensitivity and annoyance

Noise sensitivity is an intervening variable between noise exposure and annoyance, which explains much of the variance between noise exposure and individual annoyance responses. In community studies of environmental noise a modest but consistent association has usually been found between noise sensitivity and noise annoyance, (Moreira & Bryan, 1972; Pearson et al. 1974; Langdon, 1976b; Weinstein, 1978; Langdon et al. 1981; Öhrström et al. 1988b; Moehler, 1988) with an overall mean correlation from 11 studies of $r = 0.3$ (Job, 1988).

Job (1988) suggests that noise exposure is not the cause of the sensitivity–annoyance association because (1) correlations between sensitivity and noise level (mean $r = 0.01$) are consistently lower than those between sensitivity and annoyance, (2) with noise exposure controlled the mean correlation between sensitivity and annoyance is still $r = 0.22$; and (3) sensitivity and noise exposure combined account for more variance in annoyance (mean $r = 0.49$) than noise exposure alone (mean $r = 0.37$). Noise sensitivity is clearly an important contributor to explaining variance in annoyance but are they measuring the same concept? Taylor (1984) vigorously justifies the independence of sensitivity from annoyance on two grounds. First, sensitivity is a distinct psychological trait which differs from annoyance and has face validity of its own. Sensitivity, he says, 'refers to a predisposition to perceive noisy events as compared with annoyance which is an attitudinal dimension indicating the extent to which noisy events are evaluated unfavourably'. Secondly, and here he is on stronger ground, if noise sensitivity and annoyance are the same then they should have similar associations with other variables. Patently, they do not. This is most pertinent for noise exposure level, which is strongly associated with annoyance but not with sensitivity. This distinction was confirmed by Raw & Griffiths (1988) who found that while annoyance levels changed with a change in community noise exposure, sensitivity did not.

Physiological correlates of noise sensitivity

The risk of contamination of subjective sensitivity by annoyance and the possibility of response bias in sensitivity related to negative attitudes towards noise sources has led to a search for more 'objective' measures of noise sensitivity. Since the work of Stephens (1970) on magnitude scaling, there have been several attempts to quantify noise sensitivity using psychophysical scaling. However, wide consistent individual differences in the slope of the loudness function (Barbenza *et al.* 1970) were not related to self-report measures of noise sensitivity, (Stephens, 1970; Anderson, 1971; Moreira & Bryan, 1972; Waddell & Gronwall, 1984) although associations between uncomfortable loudness level (ULL) and noise sensitivity have been found (Thomas & Jones, 1982). Similarly, Öhrström *et al.* (1988*b*) found small correlations between discomfort thresholds for sound ($r = 0.27$) and cold ($r = 0.1$) and annoyance to taped traffic noise.

Auditory stimulus sensitivity, a technique for assessing pain behaviour, developed for use in migraine patients (of whom 90 % report noise to

be the most frequently avoided stimulus), has been related to a general sensitivity scale and correlated with changes in mean temporal artery blood volume in response to noise exposure (Phillips & Hunter, 1982; Rojahn & Gerhards, 1986).

If noise sensitivity identifies a group vulnerable to the effects of noise then it would be expected that noise sensitive people might exhibit a different pattern of physiological reactivity to noise. A seminal study in this area was that of Atherley *et al.* (1970) who found that the ranking of the subjective importance of a series of sounds (crying baby, alarm bell ringing, jet aircraft taxing, white noise) correlated with the length of the decay time of the skin resistance response to these sounds. Similarly a study of dental engine noise (Gang & Teft, 1975) also suggests an association between the importance of the meaning of the sound and the magnitude of the physiological response.

In these studies physiological reactions have been associated with the meaning of sounds rather than noise sensitivity in general. It may be that noise sensitivity is not specific enough and that the meaning of different sounds for individuals has a more powerful effect on psychophysiological reactivity than a general measure of reactivity to all noise. Noise sensitivity measured by Bregman and Pearson's Noise Annoyance Sensitivity Scale has been significantly associated with failure of habituation of the vasoconstriction response to noise measured by finger plethysmography (Cohen *et al.* 1973). Di Nisi *et al.* (1987), however, found no differences in finger pulse amplitude between extreme groups of high and low sensitive men and women exposed to a range of noises in the laboratory but did find that the high sensitive group demonstrated a higher average heart rate response. Rövekamp (1983) also demonstrated raised heart rate in sensitive subjects exposed to noise but his choice of sample was highly selected. There has been little other work examining the psychophysiological correlates of noise sensitivity except Ising *et al.*'s (1980) study where noise sensitivity questionnaire scores were associated with increased heart rate and blood pressure in response to a day-long exposure to taped traffic noise of 85dBA. The earlier community study of women living in West London showed unexpectedly that tonic heart rate was slower for highly sensitive women (Stansfeld et al. 1985b). In summary, the psychophysiological correlates of noise sensitivity are inconsistent.

Noise sensitivity and general sensitivity

It is vital to discover whether noise sensitivity is either part of a general reaction to a wide range of environmental stimuli or is specific to noise. If it is specific to noise this would support the case for an underlying mechanism for noise sensitivity located within the auditory system, whereas an association between noise sensitivity and general sensitivity would be more in favour of a mechanism associated with constitutional factors.

Noise annoyance (NA), in fact, a measure of noise sensitivity, on the Broadbent Gregory Noise Annoyance Scale shows a fairly strong association with general annoyance, ($r = 0.57$, $P < 0.001$ (Broadbent, 1972); $r = 0.72$ $P < 0.001$ (Anderson, 1971); $r = 0.51$ $P < 0.01$ (Weinstein, 1978); $r = 0.64$ $P < 0.001$ (Thomas & Jones, 1982). This suggests that individuals who are annoyed by noise are likely to be annoyed by other aspects of the environment. This is supported by my findings in a follow-up study of 77 women of high and low noise sensitivity living in either high aircraft noise areas around Heathrow airport and low noise areas where there was a significant correlation ($r = 0.34$–0.56) between noise sensitivity and general sensitivity (Stansfeld et al. 1985a) and by Öhrström et al. (1988b) that discomfort thresholds for intensity of sound, light and temperature were significant correlated ($r = 0.25$–0.52) in a sample of university students. Jonnson (1964) found that subjects who were troubled by noise were also troubled by air pollution and Broadbent (1972) showed that subjects scoring highly on noise annoyance showed a general negativity and were less favourably disposed to food, holidays and beauty. Such negativity towards the environment is reflected in studies of locus of control and noise annoyance (Thomas & Jones, 1982; Aniansson et al. 1983), suggesting that individuals with external locus of control were more annoyed by noise than those with internal locus of control. It might be argued that their noise annoyance scores tend to reflect their preoccupation with external events and that they may find noise particularly troublesome because they feel themselves to be at the mercy of environmental events. Noise sensitive subjects may considers themselves victims of their environment rather than in control of it, which would fit with Glass & Singer's experiments (1972) which found that subjects lacking 'perceived control' over noise exposure showed greater noise aftereffects.

Weinstein (1980) sees this rather differently, hypothesizing noise sensitivity as part of a critical-uncritical dimension, which showed the same association as noise sensitivity, to measures of noise, privacy, air pollution and neighbourhood reactions. He suggests that the most critical subjects, among whom noise sensitive subjects would be grouped, are not uniformly negative about their environment but are more discriminating than the uncritical group who comment uniformly on their environment. Langdon (1976c) would agree, suggesting that those who are not sensitive to noise are less responsive than noise sensitive people to decline in environmental quality. It is not clear from this work whether noise sensitivity is either an index of greater awareness of noxious influences in the environment or an index of general complaint.

Noise sensitivity and personality

If noise sensitivity measures a supposedly stable responsivity to noise, can it be explained in terms of conventional personality dimensions? Work relating noise sensitivity and personality has given rise to contradictory results, related to the wide variety of tests used, the poverty of the noise sensitivity measures (Griffiths & Delauzun, 1977) the unrepresentative nature of the samples studied (Moreira & Bryan, 1972) and the conditions under which testing has been carried out. Despite all these study disadvantages some common themes emerge: particularly an association between noise sensitivity and neuroticism, (Anderson, 1971; Thomas & Jones, 1982; Öhrström et al. 1988b; Jelinkova, 1988), although not all studies have found this association (Broadbent, 1972). Keshavan et al. (1981) found that noise intolerance as a prominent symptom of post-traumatic syndrome following closed head injury was more closely associated with pre-traumatic neuroticism assessed by relatives than with objective degree of trauma.

In addition, associations have been found between introversion and noise sensitivity (Fuller & Robinson, 1973; Weinstein, 1978; Thomas & Jones, 1982) but these have not been consistent (Anderson, 1971).

These findings are similar to Weinstein's study (1978) of three student samples where he found that noise sensitive individuals showed a desire for privacy, were annoyed by common annoyances, were less comfortable in social situations, and were lower in dominance, capacity for status, sociability and social presence. They were also considered less intellectually able, and less able to work persistently. This latter finding accords with his longitudinal study of students where those who were more disturbed by noise tended to have ranked lower in school classes. Thus, there are some consistencies in this personality research: there seems to be an association between noise sensitivity and neuroticism and between noise sensitivity and sensitivity to other aspects of the environment although this association has not always been found, and the nature of the association still needs further elucidation.

Noise sensitivity and psychiatric disorder

As well as associations with personality questionnaire scores such as neuroticism, noise sensitivity has also been related to current psychiatric disorder. Bennett (1945) found that annoyance to a range of different noise sources, in fact, sensitivity to noise, discriminated between a group of neurotic army personnel and a surgically and medically hospitalized control group. More recent community studies have shown (Tarnopolsky *et al.* 1978; Tarnopolsky & Morton-Williams, 1980) that noise sensitivity was significantly associated with psychiatric disorder measured by the 30-item General Health Questionnaire where 36% of more sensitive, 20% of same sensitive and 19% of less sensitive respondents were high GHQ scorers (scoring 5 or more). This association did not reveal either the type of disorder involved or the strength of the association with psychiatric 'caseness'. A further study (Stansfeld *et al.* 1985*a*) on a subset of high and low noise sensitive women living either in high noise areas around Heathrow airport or low aircraft noise areas in West London found that high noise

sensitivity was particularly associated with phobic disorders and neurotic depression measured by the Present State Examination (Wing *et al.* 1974).

A similar association has been reported in Japan using a Weinstein's sensitivity scale and the Cornell Medical Index (Iwata, 1984), suggesting that this association transcends cultural factors. Similarly, Pocnaru *et al.* (1987) showed high rates of anxiety, depression and phobias, more sleep disturbance and greater use of tranquillisers among 30 'complainers' about noise than among 30 control subjects living in the same environment; however, there may have been self-selection for ill health in this study. Similar to this association with phobic symptoms, noise sensitivity has also been linked to a coping style based on avoidance (Pulles *et al.* 1988).

Not only has an association with current psychiatric disorder been found, but Nyström and Lindegård (1975) reported that noise sensitivity as one of a group of 'asthenic subclinical symptoms' predicted the later occurrence of largely depressive illness in a prospective longitudinal study of 3019 Norwegian men. This was a tentative finding because only a single item was used to measure noise sensitivity and the correlation was small. The association was not significant when only a small 'nuclear' group of those without a previous history of psychiatric disorder was considered.

From quite a different perspective, Carman (1973) reported a small sample of patients with severe depressive illness who were hyperacusic and responded well to imipramine. He proposed that hyperacusis might be a biological marker for central serotoninergic hypoactivity. This suggests a different mechanism specific to the auditory system. It is not clear that hyperacusis is the same as noise sensitivity.

In summary, noise exposure level is related to noise annoyance, but not to psychiatric disorder. Nevertheless, noise annoyance is related to psychiatric disorder. The most potent predictor of noise annoyance, apart from noise level, is noise sensitivity which is also associated with psychiatric disorder (Fig. 1). The question then arises is noise sensitivity a predictive risk factor for psychiatric disorder or is it secondary to existing psychiatric illness? Secondly, is noise

S. A. Stansfeld

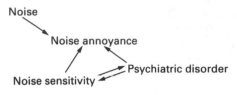

FIG. 1. Noise, sensitivity and psychiatric disorder.

THE STUDIES

Two studies are described in the monograph examining the question of whether noise sensitivity is either a predictor or a risk factor for psychiatric disorder. The first study examines the stability of noise sensitivity, and its power as a predictor of psychiatric disorder. The second study examines change in noise sensitivity with change in depression over time in depressed patients and matched control subjects and investigates the psychophysiological correlates of depression in a sub-sample.

sensitivity, as such a risk factor, a stable personality characteristic? Thirdly, is there any evidence that noise sensitivity is associated with vulnerability to noise exposure measured by psychophysiological indices?

Study 1

METHOD

If noise sensitivity was found to be a stable trait then the association between noise sensitivity and current psychiatric disorder might be the result of psychiatric disorder occurring more frequently in individuals who were already noise sensitive. Thus, highly noise sensitive people might be more prone to develop psychiatric disorder than less noise sensitive people.

As the earlier study (Stansfeld *et al.* 1985 a) had provided copious data on the 77 women interviewed, both from 1977 when they were originally interviewed and 1980 when they were interviewed again, it was felt that interviewing these women again three years later, using a postal survey would be an economical way of asking these questions in a preliminary fashion. This provided data on noise sensitivity, psychiatric disorder, and annoyance on these 77 women for three different points in time, each three years apart. The procedure involved follow-up of women interviewed three years earlier (Stansfeld *et al.* 1985 a) who were still living in areas of high and low aircraft noise exposure.

Hypothesis 1 Noise sensitivity is a stable trait and noise sensitivity scores remain stable over the three occasions of testing.

Hypothesis 2 Noise sensitivity predisposes to the later development of psychiatric morbidity. Women who are highly noise sensitive on the first occasion of testing will be more likely to exhibit psychiatric morbidity (as measured by the General Health Questionnaire) on the two second occasions of testing than women who are of low sensitivity to noise.

Sample

Subjects were drawn from the sample of 6000 individuals living in West London who were included in the West London Survey of Aircraft Noise and Psychiatric Morbidity (Tarnopolsky & Morton Williams, 1980). This random sample was distributed over much of West London and was stratified into two major zones of differing aircraft noise exposure using the Noise and Number Index (NNI), a measure of aircraft noise devised and measured by the Civil Aviation Authority and consisting of perceived noise intensity in decibels and frequency of exposure to aircraft noise. The high noise zone close to Heathrow Airport was exposed to greater than 45 NNI, while the peripheral low noise zone was exposed to less than 45 NNI.

Subjects

In 1980 women between the age of 18 and 50 years from the original West London Survey sample in 1977 were chosen, excluding those who were not born in the United Kingdom and those with gross hearing impairment. Subjects were chosen from two groups: those who were (*a*) highly sensitive and (*b*) low sensitive on both the 'McKennell' and 'Self-Report' noise sensitivity measures in 1977. These 77 subjects were followed up by postal questionnaire. As previously, subjects were contacted by Social and Community Planning Research, an independent survey organization, asking for their cooperation in a study of health and the environment.

Questionnaire

The questionnaire began with a general question about the subjects' health and several questions about reactions to the environment. These were followed by the Self-Report and McKennell noise sensitivity measures which were modified from interview administered questions to self report questionnaire form (Stansfeld *et al.* 1985 a) and questions on annoyance relating specifically to aircraft and traffic noise. The health measure comprised the 30-item General Health Questionnaire. Finally, there were 20 items from the Cognitive Failures Questionnaire (CFQ) (Broadbent *et al.* 1982) included as part of a collaborative project (Smith & Stansfeld, 1986).

Postal survey

The questionnaire, with an introductory letter, was sent out to all subjects. Those subjects who did not reply were sent a reminder letter and then, if no reply was obtained, a further letter and questionnaire. A small number of non-respondents were then followed up by telephone reminder and personal delivery of further questionnaires.

RESULTS

Seventy-seven respondents from 1980 were sent questionnaires in 1983. Sixteen respondents had moved and were thus excluded from the study and one respondent refused to complete the questionnaire. Thirty-nine replies were gathered from the first request, twelve replies after the second and third requests, five after telephone follow-up and a further four after a personal visit. The overall response rate was 78%. There was a trend towards highly noise sensitive women moving house more than less sensitive women between 1980 and 1983 but this occurred equally in high and low noise areas and respondents did not differ in marital status, age, or home ownership between noise areas in 1983.

Stability of noise sensitivity and annoyance measures

McKennell noise sensitivity scores in 1977 were highly significantly correlated with McKennell scores in 1980, and the 1980 scores likewise with the 1983 scores (Table 1) 'High' noise sensitivity was more stable than 'low' noise sensitivity. A similar pattern was observed for the Self-Report Scale though the correlations were smaller. This may relate either to the small range of values for the Self-Report scale (0–4) as opposed to the McKennell scale or may be result from poorer

repeatability for the Self-Report scale. Annoyance from aircraft noise showed similar high correlations from 1977 to 1980, and 1980 and 1983 but correlations between annoyance from 'other' sources of noise was less consistent.

Noise sensitivity as a predictor of noise annoyance

The correlations between aircraft noise annoyance in 1980 and 1983 for those who were either high or low sensitive in 1977 is shown in Table 2. Those subjects who were high sensitive in 1977 were more consistently annoyed between 1980 and 1983 than those who were low sensitive in 1977. High sensitive subjects in 1977 also had higher mean annoyance scores in 1980 and 1983 for aircraft noise, traffic noise, and other noise (Table 3). When this was examined according to aircraft noise exposure, high noise sensitive subjects demonstrated significantly higher noise annoyance in high noise but not in low noise areas (Table 4).

Table 2. *Correlations between annoyance scores in 1980 and 1983 for women either low or high sensitivity to noise in 1977.*

	High sensitivity (N = 32) r	Low sensitivity (N = 28) r
Annoyance from aircraft noise, 1980/83	0·85	0·32
Annoyance from traffic noise, 1980/83	0·51	0·30
Annoyance from other noise, 1980/83	0·51	0·23

Table 1. *Spearman correlation coefficients for noise sensitivity and noise annoyance for two three-year periods*

	McKennell sensitivity r	Self-report sensitivity r	Annoyance Aircraft noise r	Traffic noise r	Other noise r
1977–1980 (N = 77)	0·66	0·58	—	—	—
1980–1983 (N = 60)	0·68	0·43	0·68	0·49	0·46

All correlations significant at P < 0·001.

Table 3. *Mean (S.D.) noise annoyance scores for aircraft, traffic and other noise in 1980 and 1983 for low and high noise sensitive women in 1977*

	Low sensitive	High sensitive
Annoyance		
Aircraft noise 1980	3·0 (2·4)	4·0 (2·4)
Aircraft noise 1983	2·5 (1·7)	4·1 (2·2)**
Traffic noise 1980	1·8 (0·3)	2·2 (0·3)**
Traffic noise 1983	2·0 (1·6)	3·5 (2·1)**
Other noise 1980	1·2 (1·9)	3·0 (2·5)***
Other noise 1983	1·6 (2·5)	4·1 (2·6)***

** P < 0·01; *** P 0·001.

Table 4. *Mean annoyance (S.D.) by aircraft noise in 1980 and 1983 according to aircraft noise exposure and noise sensitivity in 1977*

	Low NS 1977		High NS 1977	
	Low noise	High noise	Low noise	High noise
1980	2·5 (2·3)	3·44 (2·1)	2·52 (2·1)	5·75 (1·5)**
1983	2·1 (1·8)	2·82 (1·7)	2·69 (2·1)	5·56 (1·5)**

** $P < 0.01$.

Noise sensitivity as a predictor of psychiatric disorder

In studying whether McKennell and Self-Report sensitivity predicted later psychiatric disorder, the General Health Questionnaire responses in 1980 and 1983 were used as the outcome variable. Respondents were defined as a 'possible case' if they scored 5 or more on the 30-item General Health Questionnaire. This threshold was chosen as giving the best sensitivity and specificity in the earlier validation study on this sample. With the availability of two years outcome data the analysis was repeated using 'possible caseness'

Table 5. *Noise sensitivity as a predictor of GHQ 'caseness'*

GHQ 1980	'Non-case'	'Case'	Total
Sensitivity in 1977 as a predictor of GHQ 'caseness' in 1980 for 52 respondents, 'non-cases' in 1977.			
Sensitivity Low	21	6 (22%)	27
1977 High	20	5 (20%)	25
Total	41	11	52

GHQ 1980/1983	'Non-case'	'Case'	Total
Sensitivity in 1977 as a predictor of GHQ 'caseness' in 1980 or 1983 for 'non-cases' in 1977			
Sensitivity Low	15	12 (44%)	27
1977 High	9	16 (64%)	25
Total	24	28	52

in either year as the outcome variable. Although there was a small excess of 'caseness' in those women who were more sensitive in 1977, this difference was non significant and again the numbers were too small for adequate testing of the hypothesis and the estimates of 'caseness' were biased by differential drop out rates (Table 5).

Study 2

METHOD

Noise sensitivity and depressive illness

After the association between noise sensitivity and psychiatric disorder, particularly depression, had been confirmed in a community sample of women (Stansfeld *et al.* 1985*a*) it seemed logical to examine noise sensitivity in a group of depressed patients for three reasons. First, if noise sensitivity is a biological marker for depressive illness it should be particularly apparent in a sample of depressed patients. Secondly, there have been intriguing clues that noise sensitivity might be associated with particular subtype of depressive illness related to a specific underlying biochemical abnormality. Thirdly, in order to examine the longitudinal course of the association between psychiatric disorder and noise sensitivity, by following changes in noise sensitivity with remission from depression it was more economic to study a group of depressed patients, as the prevalence of depression, particularly severe depression, is small in a community samples. The second study, which included a pilot study, examined noise sensitivity scores in a depressed population and a group of non-depressed age and sex-matched control subjects. This study aimed to discover whether noise sensitive depressed patients constituted an identifiable subgroup of depressive illness in terms of symptoms, personality and physiological responsivity. It also aimed to determine whether patients who were noise sensitive while depressed became less noise sensitive as they recovered from depression. Noise sensitivity scores were measured on two occasions: in depressed patients, when they were acutely ill and four months later when a proportion had recovered from depression. This strategy was used to adduce evidence for a state-dependent component of noise sensitivity.

Following the pilot study where noise sensitivity in depressed patients did not seem to alter over time (for further details see Stansfeld, 1989), noise sensitivity was also assessed in an age and sex matched group of non-depressed control subjects with the aim of assessing whether there was an absolute difference in noise sensitivity between depressed patients and normal subjects.

Hypothesis 1 There is a subgroup of severely depressed patients who are highly sensitive to noise. These noise sensitive patients differ in symptoms, personality and physiological responsivity from other depressed patients.

Hypothesis 2 Highly noise sensitive depressed patients become less noise sensitive as they recover from depression.

Hypothesis 3 In the laboratory highly noise sensitive subjects will habituate more slowly to a threatening noise (drill noise) than low noise sensitive subjects, but habituation of subjects to non-threatening noise (pure tones) will not be affected by their noise sensitivity.

A pilot study was carried out before embarking on Study 2. It did not decisively settle the question of whether noise sensitivity varied with intensity of depression but it clarified the choice of suitable instruments, suggested that a longer period of follow-up would be suitable before retesting for noise sensitivity and found that a larger sample would be necessary to find enough highly noise sensitive subjects (Stansfeld, 1989). In addition, because the pilot study indicated that noise sensitivity was very stable over time and might be considered a trait, it seemed important to test whether, in this sample, noise sensitivity differed between depressed patients and non-depressed control subjects. The objective of the study was to examine the noise sensitivity of a depressed patient population, both during depressive illness and following recovery. The association between noise sensitivity and clinical subtypes of depressive illness, personality measures and physiological responsivity were also examined. A control group of non-depressed subjects was also included to assess any differences in noise sensitivity between these subjects and depressed patients.

Experimental design

The experiment included (*a*) a cross-sectional comparison of noise sensitivity within depressed patients, (*b*) a prospective follow-up study of depressed patients, and (*c*) a cross-sectional and prospective comparison of depressed patients with a matched control group of normal subjects.

Selection of study population

Depressed patients were selected from in-patients and out-patients at the Maudsley and Bethlem Royal Hospitals, King's College Hospital, St Giles' Hospital and Farnborough Hospital. All the hospitals serve catchment areas within south east London, although Farn-borough Hospital takes patients primarily from the suburbs on the south east border of London.

Selection criteria

(*a*) Depressed patients

Depressed patients were included who fulfilled the Research Diagnostic Criteria (Spitzer *et al.* 1978) for either major or minor depressive disorder. Patients with other primary psychiatric diagnoses were excluded. Men and women between the ages of 18 and 65 years were eligible for inclusion. Patients with gross clinical deafness were excluded although data were collected on patients with milder degrees of deafness for use as a comparison group in the main study.

(*b*) Control subjects

Control subjects were selected from among Institute of Psychiatry, Maudsley Hospital and King's College Hospital staff who were unaware of the study hypotheses. Subjects were matched for sex and age (within one year) with depressed patients. Two further criteria needed to be fulfilled before control subjects were matched with depressed patients; first, that control subjects had never suffered from clinical depressive illness and, secondly, that they had normal hearing.

Data collection

Initially, data were collected by interview of depressed patients. Follow-up data on depressed patients were obtained by postal questionnaire. The interview comprised a standardized psychiatric interview to measure depression, a self completion symptom questionnaire to act as a baseline for measuring change in depression and two noise sensitivity questionnaires. The order of questionnaires was counterbalanced although in the noise sensitivity sections the Weinstein Noise Sensitivity Scale (Weinstein, 1978) always followed the Broadbent–Gregory General Annoyance Questionnaire (Broadbent, 1972; Anderson, 1971). In the latter questionnaire the noise items are disguised by their insertion among many general annoyance items, while the former questionnaire is clearly directed towards noise. The fixed order of the noise sensitivity questionnaires was chosen so as to keep the specific interest of the study in noise hidden as much as possible from patients while completing the Broadbent–Gregory General Annoyance Questionnaire.

Measurement of depression

The Present State Examination (PSE), a structured psychiatric interview (Wing, *et al.* 1974) was used to measure depressive illness. This instrument has the advantage of being designed to measure severe psychiatric illness, particularly psychotic illness and was therefore suitable for many of the more severely ill subjects in this sample. It has several further advantages over an observer-rated measure of depression such as the Hamilton Depression Rating Scale (Hamilton, 1967). The criteria for scoring symptoms are more clearly defined in the PSE and use of the interview and its scoring system are standardized by a training course which is not required for the Hamilton Rating Scale. (The interviewer who was originally trained in the use of the PSE in 1980 was also able to re-standardize his clinical evaluations by scoring videotaped interviews at the MRC Social Psychiatry Unit.) The PSE also provides useful output for comparisons between different clinical sub-populations of depression. The simplest measures are those of Total Symptom scores and subscores. In addition, it groups symptoms into diagnostic subclasses and classes and, through the CATEGO program, provides diagnoses according to the eighth edition of the International Classification of Diseases. Finally, it also gives a measurement of the certainty that the patient is a 'case' of psychiatric disorder through the 'Index of Definition'.

Symptom Rating Test

This 30-item self-completion questionnaire (SRT) (Kellner & Sheffield, 1973) was chosen to measure change in symptom scores for depressed patients between the two occasions of testing and, secondly, to act as a screening questionnaire for control subjects to exclude those with current depression. It has been used widely to measure symptom scores in depressed patients and has been shown particularly sensitive to change. A total score and four subscale scores are obtainable from the questionnaire. The scales are Depression (8 items), Anxiety (8 items), Somatic (7 items) and Inadequacy (7 items). In order to be relevant to the current state of the patient the weekly version was used in which patients are asked to describe how they have felt during the past week.

Measurement of noise sensitivity

Broadbent–Gregory Annoyance Questionnaire

This is a 40-item questionnaire which yields two subscales, that of noise annoyance, in fact a measure of noise sensitivity (NA) (10 items), and general annoyance (GA) (30 items) (Broadbent, 1972). The 10 noise items were left unchanged from the original questionnaire but the general annoyance items were updated to make them more relevant to the current concerns of subjects. Subjects are asked to rate their annoyance on a four-point scale from 'not annoying' to 'extremely annoying'. As 'state' annoyance response rather than 'trait' annoyance response was sought subjects were asked 'During the last week, how annoying would you have found the following things and situations if they had happened?'. Thus, subjects were instructed to report their annoyance responses for the same time period as their symptoms responses on the SRT. The disadvantage of this procedure was that many subjects had not experienced any of these potentially annoying situations during the last week. Some of their responses were, therefore, undoubtedly supposition as to how they *would have* reacted rather than memories of how they *had* reacted. This mode of response was not a problem to most subjects but may have tended to encourage 'trait' rather than 'state' responses. Cronbach's alpha coefficient was 0·82 for the NA scale in depressed patients.

Weinstein Noise Sensitivity Scale

This is a series of 21 statements relating to noise sensitivity with which subjects are asked to state their agreement or disagreement on a 6-point scale from 'agree strongly' to 'disagree strongly' (Weinstein, 1978). Minor changes in wording were made which have the agreement of the original author in order for the questionnaire to be suitable for British rather than North American subjects. The Kuder–Richardson (Richardson & Kuder, 1939) reliability coefficient was 0·76 in depressed patients.

Psychophysiological measurements on depressed patients and control subjects

This section of the study aimed to demonstrate psychophysiological responsivity to noise in noise sensitive, as opposed to less sensitive subjects, especially in terms of delayed habituation to unpleasant noise. It was anticipated that the small differences expected might be easier to demonstrate in the controlled conditions of the laboratory than they had been in the field in the earlier study (Stansfeld *et al.* 1985*b*).

If tonic differences in heart rate and skin conductance were probably subject to substantial random error through measurement in the community study, then perhaps tonic differences might be demonstrated in the more carefully controlled conditions of the laboratory. In addition, as both state and tonic levels of skin conductance and heart rate showed little conclusive in the West London Study (Stansfeld *et al.* 1985*b*), then it might be that the wrong variables were being measured. If noise sensitive individuals found it more difficult to adapt to noise exposure than less sensitive individuals it is possible that noise sensitive individuals would habituate to noise more slowly than less sensitive individuals.

There are factors both from within the individual e.g. mood, personality, which contribute to noise sensitivity and might contribute to individual differences in physiological responsivity, and factors related to the noise itself such as loudness, and impulsiveness. From a cognitive view point the 'meaning' of the noise may well be important for the individual and people may report themselves as sensitive to noises which carry important information for them. In particular, if noises are noxious or threatening people might be expected to report that they are more upset or annoyed by these noises. In psychophysiological measurements such noises might be expected to elicit an orientating reflex or even startle/defence reflexes, particularly in those reporting noise sensitivity. Moreover, these reflexes may be expected to be more evident in response to noises generally held to be noxious or aversive such as 'drill' noise rather than in response to probably neutral sounds such as pure tones. In this part of Study 2 the habituation rate to a series of pure tones and road drill noise is examined.

Selection of subjects

Patients suffering from primary depressive disorder (according to RDC for either major or minor depressive disorder) who were either in patients or out-patients at the Bethlem Royal and Maudsley Hospital were tested. They were between 18 and 60 years of age and of both sexes. They were of normal hearing, as tested by audiometry.

Control subjects, without history of psychiatric disorder, were selected to be matched for age and sex with the depressed patients. They were also of normal hearing for their age group. The upper age limit of 65 years chosen for the main study was lowered to reduce the possibility of including any subjects with minor degrees of hearing impairment.

Psychophysiological study procedure

Pre-test instructions More details of the procedure, including electrode placement, tone and drill noise generation are to be found in Stansfeld (1989). Subjects were seated in the laboratory ante-room and asked to complete the Bond–Lader scale (Bond *et al.* 1974) a state mood questionnaire. After the electrodes had been attached they were seated in the laboratory and told they would hear a series of noises through the headphones. Approximately 10 min elapsed between the subjects entry to the laboratory and the start of testing.

Attachment of electrodes Heart-rate electrodes were attached to the dorsal surface of both forearms. The active skin conductance electrode was attached to the volar surface of the terminal

phalanx of the (L) thumb positioned over the central whorl of the thumb print.

Experimental design Each subject heard a series of 18 presentations of a pure tone and 18 presentations of pneumatic drill noise through the headphones. Half the subjects heard the tones first and half the subjects heard the drill noise first. The tones and the drill noise were matched for intensity, duration and rise time. The sounds (tones and drill noise) were of three intensities 50 dBA, 75 dBA and 100 dBA. The sounds were divided into six triplets of 50, 75, 100 db intensity. These triplets consisted of the six possible orders of presentation of the three sounds. The triplets were presented in a random order which was fixed for all subjects. Each sound lasted for 4 s. The sounds were enclosed in an envelope of 30 ms rise time and 30 ms declination. The tones were of 1 kHz frequency and the drill noises were naturally, of mixed frequency although the lowest frequencies were excluded by the recording technique. There was a random interval of between 30 and 50 s, between sounds. These intervals were fixed for all subjects. The series of tones immediately followed the series of noises (and vice versa).

Apparatus

Physiological recording Heart-rate recordings were processed to provide second-by-second mean interbeat interval scores for 5 s before the onset of the sound and 10 s after the onset of the sound. There was a continuous record of skin conductance on polygraph paper throughout the period of listening to the sounds.

Scoring of electrodermal activity prestimulus skin resistance levels Tonic skin resistance was measured prior to each response deflection of each of the 36 stimuli and converted to skin conductance.

Skin conductance responses Skin conductance responses were considered as having been evoked by the stimulus if they were greater than 0·02 micromhos and occurred between 1 and 5 s after stimulus onset. Skin conductance responses were: the log pre-stimulus skin conductance level minus the log post-stimulus skin conductance level at peak amplitude.

Scoring of heart rate   Heart rate was measured as interbeat interval for 5 s before the stimulus and for 10 s after the stimulus. An overall mean prestimulus value was calculated as the mean of the five prestimulus scores. The 10 post-stimulus scores were expressed as difference scores from the overall prestimulus mean score.

Missing data on heart rate   The heart-rate programme recognized interbeat interval values greater than 1310 as missing data. Twenty-seven such values were recognized in the total heart rate data for the 36 subjects (i.e. 5 %). Missing data were found in 9 of the 36 subjects. In order to run repeated measures analyses these missing data were replaced with estimated values. If the missing value occurred at the end of a record then the previous value was substituted.

Post-test assessment

The subjects were first asked whether they could identify the drill noise sound and were asked to write down their answer. This was followed by a semantic differential scale of 13 adjective pairs, derived from Anderson's Noise Specific Annoyance Questionnaire in which subjects were asked about the loudest of the series of noises. This scale measures how annoying the noise is for subjects. Then subjects were asked whether they had been more or less sensitive to noise than usual recently and finally they completed a further state mood scale.

RESULTS

General characteristics of the patient sample

One hundred and thirty-five patients were interviewed over 10 months. Eight patients were asked but refused to be interviewed. The patients were in-patients from the Maudsley, Bethlem Royal, Farnborough and St Giles' hospitals, and out-patients from the Maudsley Hospital (see Table 6).

Exclusion of subjects

Two patients were excluded from the initial 135 patients; one because the interview was not completed and one because her age was subsequently discovered to be above the age limit for the study. Ten patients were also excluded because the diagnosis was not that of primary depressive illness. This diagnosis was derived by

Table 6. *Clincial characteristics of depressed patients in Study 2*

Hospital	Maudsley	Bethlem Royal	Farnborough	St Giles
Site of patient interviews				
In-patients	46	44	26	6
Out-patients	13	—	—	—
	Hypomania 296.1	Depressive psychosis 296.2	Retarded depression 296.2/300.4	Paranoid psychosis 297.9	Depressive neurosis 300.4
ICD diagnoses (according to CATEGO program)				
2	17	82	1	21

combining their current PSE-CATEGO diagnosis and their Syndrome Check List (SCL) diagnosis for past episodes according to the guidelines laid down by the MRC Social Psychiatry Unit (Wing & Sturt, 1978). This left 123 patients who will be called the 'depressed sample'. Thirty-one patients indicated hearing impairment but were not excluded because they did not differ in noise sensitivity from patients who indicated normal hearing. Diagnoses according to the *current* PSE-CATEGO program for the depressed samples are displayed in Table 6. The distribution of Broadbent–Gregory NA scores and Weinstein NS scores is reported elsewhere (Stansfeld, 1989).

Follow-up of depressed patients

One patient from the initial 133 patients refused to take part in the follow-up examination. From the 132 patients who were sent follow-up questionnaires four months after the initial interview, 111 patients returned questionnaires resulting in a response rate of 84 %. Of those questionnaires returned, three were damaged or incomplete.

Control subjects

Eighty-two depressed patients were matched for sex and age (± 1 year) with control subjects who comprised 27 men and 55 women. Seventy-five of these control subjects also completed and returned follow-up questionnaires after 4 months.

Demographic comparisons of depressed patients and matched controls

There were no significant differences between

the 82 depressed patients and their (age and sex) matched controls for marital status (married, single, widowed/divorced/separated), and the Registrar General Social Class either for the subject themselves or the head of household. Often the problem with using staff controls may be social class differences between patients and controls but this was not the case in this study.

Noise annoyance, general annoyance and noise sensitivity

NA is moderately correlated with NS on both the first and second occasions of testing among depressed patients (see Table 7). GA is more strongly associated with NA than with NS. The correlation between NS and NA is greater than the correlation between NS and GA on both occasions of testing in both samples. Thus, although part of noise sensitivity may be accounted for by general annoyance reactions there is also a specific reaction to noise.

Despite the improvement in psychiatric state between the first and second occasions of testing for 55% of depressed patients who returned questionnaires, the correlations between the measures of NA, NS and GA on first and second occasions are high and tend to be higher than the agreement between the individual measures, excepting NA (Table 7). The results for control

subjects are fairly similar (Table 7); both NA and NS are stable in a manner similar to depressed patients over both occasions of testing although GA seems less stable in control subjects.

Noise sensitivity and hearing impairment

There were no significant differences in either NS or NA between those with normal hearing and those with impaired hearing according to audiometric thresholds for left ear alone, right ear alone and both ears combined. Impaired hearing was defined as a mean threshold greater than 25 dBA over eight frequencies from 0.5 to 8 kHz. Also hearing impairment, as measured by a direct question asking about problems with hearing, did not affect noise sensitivity in depressed patients. Mean noise annoyance scores did not differ significantly between those with 'normal' hearing (mean = 17.78, S.D. = 6.40, $N = 92$) and those with hearing impairment (mean = 17.29, S.D. = 6.92, $N = 31$, $t = -0.36$). Mean noise sensitivity scores did not differ significantly between those with normal hearing (mean = 68.21, S.D. = 14.01, $t = -0.56$) and those with hearing impairment. The depressed patients with 'normal' hearing did not differ significantly from the hearing-impaired sample in terms of severity of disorder measured by PSE

Table 7. *Spearman correlations between noise annoyance, general annoyance and noise sensitivity*

	NA 1	GA 1	NS 1	NA 2	GA 2
Depressed sample					
GA 1	0·64*** ($N = 122$)				
NS 1	0·55*** ($N = 121$)	0·36*** ($N = 120$)			
NA 2	0·62*** ($N = 102$)	0·43*** ($N = 101$)	0·48*** ($N = 100$)		
GA 2	0·47*** ($N = 102$)	0·67*** ($N = 101$)	0·28** ($N = 100$)	0·71*** ($N = 102$)	
NS 2	0·42*** ($N = 97$)	0·27** ($N = 96$)	0·67*** ($N = 95$)	0·66*** ($N = 96$)	0·42*** ($N = 96$)
Control sample					
GA 1	0·64*** ($N = 82$)				
NS 1	0·50*** ($N = 78$)	0·38*** ($N = 78$)			
NA 2	0·64*** ($N = 75$)	0·27* ($N = 75$)	0·38*** ($N = 71$)		
GA 2	0·32*** ($N = 75$)	0·41*** ($N = 75$)	0·21* ($N = 71$)	0·63*** ($N = 75$)	
NS 2	0·47*** ($N = 74$)	0·17 ($N = 74$)	0·69*** ($N = 70$)	0·64*** ($N = 74$)	0·35*** ($N = 74$)

* $P < 0.05$; ** $P < 0.01$; *** $P < 0.001$.

Table 8. *Mean noise annoyance, general annoyance and noise sensitivity scores for depressed patients and control subjects by sex*

	Women (N = 79)	Men (N = 44)	t
Depressed			
NA	17·77	17·45	0·26
GA	57·05	54·73	0·80
NS	67·76	67·91	−0·06
Control			
NA	13·15	13·04	0·06
GA	42·30	47·00	−1·55
NS	57·21	56·00	0·31

All *P* values were non-significant.

total symptom score (means 34·25, 35·84, S.D. = 10·63, 12·83, *t* = 0·68). Thus, there was no evidence that the hearing-impaired patients differed from the normal hearing patients either in terms of noise sensitivity or severity of illness.

Noise sensitivity scores did not differ significantly between men and women in either the depressed patient or the control sample (Table 8).

Noise sensitivity and depression

It was postulated that severely depressed patients are highly sensitive to noise and differ in symptoms from other depressed patients. Noise sensitivity was associated with the total number of symptoms: both NA and NS at first testing were significantly correlated with the Present State Examination Total Symptom score in the depressed sample (see Table 9). Contrary to the hypothesis, which suggested that noise-sensitive patients would be those who were severely depressed, noise-sensitive patients in this study display significantly more neurotic symptoms (as measured by the Present State Examination non-specific neurotic symptoms score) and are not those who are more severely depressed. The relationship and severity of depression was also

examined by examining Symptom Rating Test scores and subscores in relation to noise sensitivity scores. No significant association was found between Sympton Rating Test scores (and subscores) and either NS or NA measures, except that noise sensitivity was just significantly associated with the inadequacy subscore for both samples. Although this latter significant finding may be coincidental, it tends to confirm the findings of the association with non-specific neurotic symptoms.

As a further way of examining whether noise sensitivity was associated with a particular subtype of depressive illness, mean noise sensitivity scores within current diagnoses and within classes and subclasses, ascertained by the PSE-CATEGO program, were compared. Against the expectation of the hypothesis, depressed patients did not differ in mean noise sensitivity scores for either CATEGO class or CATEGO ICD-8 diagnoses (see Table 10). There was also

Table 10. *Mean noise annoyance, noise sensitivity and general annoyance scores for PSE CATEGO classes and diagnoses in depressed patients*

	R Retarded depression (N = 83) Mean (S.D.)	D Depressive psychosis (N = 19) Mean (S.D.)	N Neurotic depression (N = 21) Mean (S.D.)
CATEGO classes			
Noise annoyance	17·58 (6·5)	18·26 (5·2)	19·18 (6·5)
Noise sensitivity	67·31 (13·6)	64·84 (8·2)	67·86 (11·3)
General annoyance	56·52 (15·6)	57·42 (13·3)	55·18 (15·8)
	Psychotic or neurotic depression Mean (S.D)	Psychotic depression Mean (S.D.)	Neurotic depression Mean (S.D.)
CATEGO diagnoses			
NA	17·41 (6·84)	18·25 (5·03)	18·76 (6·3)
NS	67·85 (14·59)	65·45 (8·43)	68·0 (11·6)
GA	56·45 (16·10)	57·3 (13·0)	53·62 (14·3)

Table 9. *Spearman correlation coefficients for noise annoyance, noise sensitivity and general annoyance with PSE neurotic and total symptom scores and Symptom Rating Test scores in depressed patients*

	SRTA	SRTD	SRTS	SRTI	SRTT	PSEN	PSET	ID
NA (N = 123)	0·13	0·09	0·12	0·12	0·12	0·23**	0·19**	0·14
NS (N = 128)	0·07	0·00	0·07	0·15*	0·07	0·21**	0·15*	0·11
GA (N = 122)	0·18*	0·22**	0·17*	0·26**	0·24**	0·36***	0·30***	0·18*

*P < 0·05; ** P < 0·01; *** P < 0·001.

no association between noise sensitivity and either duration of illness measured in weeks, or number of previous episodes.

General annoyance and depression

GA has weak but significant associations, not only with PSE total symptom score and PSE non-specific neurotic symptom scores but also with the total Symptom Rating Test score and all four subscores (see Table 10). Unlike depressed subjects, there were significant associations between all symptom rating test subscales and NA, NS and GA scales scores in control subjects. On the whole, the size of the

Table 11. *Spearman correlation coefficients for noise annoyance, noise sensitivity and general annoyance with Symptom Rating Test scores in control subjects*

Noise sensitivity	Symptom Rating Test				
	SRTA	SRTD	SRTS	SRTI	SRTT
NA1 ($N = 81$)	0·26**	0·22*	0·34***	0·29**	0·35***
NA2 ($N = 74$)	0·25*	0·26*	0·35***	0·36***	0·36***
NS1 ($N = 77$)	0·23*	0·23*	0·22*	0·43***	0·35***
NS2 ($N = 73$)	0·24**	0·28**	0·20⁺	0·39***	0·32**
GA1 ($N = 81$)	0·31**	0·36***	0·33***	0·30**	0·45***
GA2 ($N = 74$)	0·25*	0·25*	0·26*	0·24*	0·29*

* $P < 0.05$; ** $P < 0.01$; *** $P < 0.001$.

Table 12. *Spearman correlation coefficients between noise sensitivity, noise annoyance and Eysenck Personality Questionnaire in depressed patients and control subjects*

	Eysenck Personality Questionnaire			
	Psychoticism	Extraversion	Neuroticism	Lie
Depressed patients				
Occasion 2				
NA	0·14	−0·06	0·29**	−0·06
($N = 96$)				
NS	0·08	−0·16	0·31***	−0·12
($N = 94$)				
GA	0·15	−0·12	0·33***	−0·01
($N = 96$)				
Control subjects				
NA1	0·08	−0·14	0·30**	−0·23*
($N = 75$)				
NS1	−0·02	−0·12	0·36***	−0·22
($N = 74$)				
GA1	0·10	−0·27*	0·32**	0·03
($N = 75$)				

* $P < 0.05$; ** $P < 0.01$; *** $P < 0.001$.

associations were quite small. It might be that they were larger than the associations within depressed patients because there was a greater heterogeneity of response within control subjects (Table 11).

Noise sensitivity and personality

It was also postulated that noise sensitive depressed patients would differ from other depressed patients, in personality as well as symptoms. This was investigated in three ways. First, NA and NS scores were correlated with scores on the three scales of the Eysenck Personality Questionnaire, completed at the same time in the follow-up questionnaire. NA, NS and GA were significantly associated with neuroticism (Table 12). This association between noise sensitivity and neuroticism confirms the findings of the earlier study (Stansfeld *et al.* 1985*a*). There were no significant associations with either introversion – extraversion, or psychoticism, or the Lie Scale. There was a trend towards an association between NS, NA, GA and introversion but this failed to reach significance. Within matched control subjects, findings were very similar, with a consistent association between NA, NS and neuroticism and generally a small negative association with both extraversion and the Lie Scale.

Secondly, mean scores for neuroticism, extraversion, psychoticism and lie scales were compared between a 'highly noise sensitive' subgroup (high NS, high NA, chosen as those more than one standard deviation above the means on either of the two noise sensitivity measures) and patients who were less noise sensitive. The 'highly noise sensitive' subgroups were not significantly different from the less noise sensitive subgroups according to these personality dimensions. Thirdly, diagnoses of personality disorder (made using the Aetiology Schedule (Wing & Sturt, 1978) after studying the patients' case note) were compared between the 'high NA' and 'high NS' subgroups and the remainder of the depressed patients. Of the 'high NA' group, five had definite personality abnormalities, insufficient to make a main diagnosis of personality disorder, (classified as anankastic, affective, hysterical, asthenic and unspecified respectively). In the 'high NS' group six had definite personality abnormalities, insufficient to make a main diagnosis of personality disorder (two were classified as asthenic, three as affective, and one hysterical).

Noise sensitivity and recovery from depression

The second hypothesis of this section of the study was that highly noise sensitive patients become less sensitive to noise as they recover from depression. The hypothesis was tested by examining the change in noise sensitivity scores for patients in the 'high NS' and 'high NA' groups between the two occasions of testing. The patients selected from these two groups had made some recovery from depression, as judged by a fall in their Symptom Rating Test total symptom scores, between the two occasions of testing. The hypothesis was confirmed in the depressed sample, in which patients from both the 'high NA' and the 'high NS' groups became significantly less noise annoyed and less noise sensitive by the second occasion of testing if their total symptom rating test scores had dropped between the first and second occasions of testing (see Table 13). It is interesting that even when highly sensitive individuals recover from depression and their noise sensitivity levels drop, these noise sensitivity levels are still high relative to the rest of the sample. This may suggest that this state variation in noise sensitivity is superimposed on an already high level of trait noise sensitivity.

Considering all patients tested on both occasions in both samples, there was a small decrease in both NA and NS between the first and second occasions of testing; this was only significant for NA in the depressed sample. This drop in NA for all patients may indicate that either a substantial proportion of patients made some recovery from depression or that lower scoring was a feature of repeated testing. It must be noted that of all patients only 55 % recovered from depression, 20 % remained similarly depressed, and 26 % became worse between the first and second occasions of testing four months apart.

It might be argued that much of the drop in NS and NA between the two occasions may be the result of 'regression to the mean'. In particular, this might explain why the sensitivity scores of high NS and high NA individuals dropped between the two occasions of testing even though the size of the drop in noise sensitivity was less than in the smaller group who made some recovery from depression. The association between change in depression scores over time and change in noise sensitivity was examined by correlating the respective change scores. There was a small statistically significant correlation between change in NA and change in depression score (to either less or more depressed), ($r = 0.20$, $P < 0.003$, $N = 101$) and between change in NS score and change in depression score ($r = 0.36$, $P < 0.001$, $N = 95$).

Noise sensitivity of depressed patients and control subjects

It was also hypothesized that depressed patients are more likely to be noise sensitive than a non-depressed control group of subjects. This hypo-

Table 13. *Comparison of mean values of noise annoyance and noise sensitivity between first and second occasions of testing in depressed patients*

	Mean noise annoyance		Difference between means	t	df
	Occasion 1	Occasion 2			
All patients	17·59	16·28	1·31*	2·24	101
Highly noise-annoyed group	27·40	23·33	4·07*	2·42	14
Highly noise-annoyed group, with drop in SRT total score	27·67	21·44	6·22*	2·58	8
	Mean noise sensitivity		Difference between means	t	df
	Occasion 1	Occasion 2			
All patients	67·75	65·50	2·25	1·98	94
Highly noise-sensitive group	88·13	82·93	5·20	1·66	14
Highly noise-sensitive group, with drop in SRT total score	87.80	78.90	8·90*	2·32	9

* $P < 0.05$.

Table 14. *Mean scores of noise annoyance, noise sensitivity and general annoyance for depressed patients and age- and sex-matched control subjects*

	Depressed patients Mean (S.D.)	Control subjects (Mean (S.D.)	*t*	*P*
NA (*N* = 82)	17·9 (6·5)	13·10 (6·0)	5·27	< 0·0001
NS (*N* = 75)	68·05 (13·6)	56·72 (15·9)	4·58	< 0·0001
GA (*N* = 81)	56·20 (14·9)	43·52 (12·7)	6·36	< 0·0001

thesis was added after the pilot study was performed, in which no change was found in noise sensitivity scores over time. It thus became imperative to test in this sample whether depressed patients differed from normal subjects in noise sensitivity. This hypothesis was strikingly confirmed for the depressed sample in comparison with sex- and age-matched (+1 year) non-depressed control subjects for both the Noise Annoyance and Weinstein Noise Sensitivity Scales (Table 14).

A further method of assessing whether depressed patients become less noise sensitive as they recover from depression was to compare the mean noise sensitivity scores of depressed patients and their matched controls, on the two occasions of testing. In particular, it seemed logical to compare the mean noise sensitivity score for (*a*) depressed patients who had made some recovery from depression between the two occasions of testing and their matched controls and (*b*) depressed patients who had either stayed similarly depressed or became worse between the two occasions of testing. Recovery from depression was defined as a lower total symptom rating test score on the second occasion of testing (group *a*), while if the symptom rating test score stayed the same or increased on the second occasion of testing they were included in group *b*.

The NA and NS scores of depressed patients whose depression improved between the two occasions of testing fell more steeply than their matched controls. For NA this presented a highly significant difference between depressive patients and control subjects at time 1 and a non-significant difference at time 2 (Table 15). This confirmed the hypothesis that depressed patients who become less depressed became less noise sensitive. For the Weinstein Scale (Table

Table 15. *Mean noise annoyance (NA) scores and Weinstein noise sensitivity (NS) scores (standard deviation) for depressed patients and matched controls at Time 1 and Time 2 for patients who (a) got better from depression, (b) stayed similarly depressed or got worse*

			Depressed patients Mean (S.D.)	Control subjects Mean (S.D.)	*t*
NA					
(a)	Better from depression				
		Time 1	17·53 (6·3)	14·16 (5·1)	3·59***
		Time 2	14·86 (6·7)	12·78 (6·1)	1·77
(b)	Stayed the same or worse on depression				
		Time 1	18·07 (7·0)	11·53 (6·2)	4·61****
		Time 2	17·39 (7·6)	11·61 (6·4)	2·22*
NA					
(a)	Better from depression				
		Time 1	67·89 (14·7)	58·77 (13·3)	3·28**
		Time 2	61·42 (16·0)	54·38 (14·1)	2·79*
(b)	Stayed the same or worse on depression				
		Time 1	68·00 (11·9)	55·15 (17·5)	3·53**
		Time 2	70·00 (15·1)	56·39 (16·1)	2·51*

* *P* < 0·05; *** *P* < 0·001; **** < 0·00001.

15) a similar pattern was observed, except that there was a significant difference between depressed patients and control subjects at time 2 as well at time 1. While part of this finding may be explained as a characteristic related to repeated testing it would also fit with the Weinstein Questionnaire measuring the trait aspects of noise sensitivity and thus not changing so much, while the NA scores, measuring state sensitivity, fell more abruptly (Fig. 2).

For those who stayed similarly depressed, or became worse, NA scores, in keeping with the hypothesis, remained fairly stable in both depressed and control groups which differed significantly from each other on both occasions of testing (Table 15). On the Weinstein Scale depressed patients actually became more noise sensitive greatly against the general trend between the two occasions of testing, and a small reverse was also noted for control subjects. Again, in accordance with the hypothesis with a maintenance or increase in depression scores, noise sensitivity scores were maintained or slightly increased and noise sensitivity scores of the depressed and control groups remained significantly different on both occasions of testing (Table 15). This contradicts the assertion

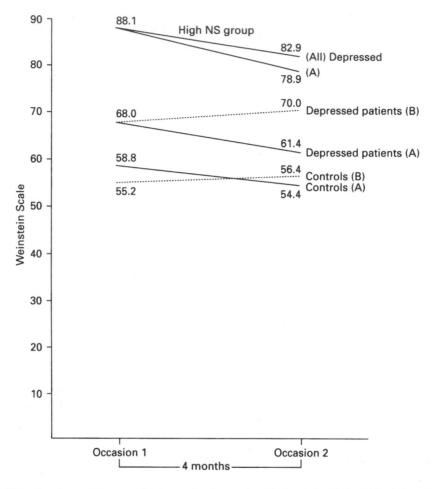

FIG. 2. Mean Weinstein noise sensitivity scores for depressed patients and matched control subjects: (A) better from depression (——); (B) same or worse from depression (····).

that the fall in noise sensitivity scores is explained totally by regression to the mean.

Psychophysiological results

Psychophysiological testing of heart rate and skin conductance was carried out in a subsample of 18 depressed patients and 18 matched control subjects in the laboratory. The results reported here are those relating directly to noise sensitivity measured on the Broadbent–Gregory (NA) scale and the Weinstein (NS) scale.

Pre-experimental skin conductance level

There were no main effects of between-subjects factors and no significant differences between both (*a*) pre-experimental and (*b*) post-exper-

imental skin conductance level in repeated measures analysis of variance.

Spontaneous response frequency

High NS subjects demonstrated more spontaneous fluctuations in pre-experiment ($F = 4.47$, df 1, 35, $P < 0.05$) and post-experiment ($F = 8.03$, df 1, 28, $P < 0.009$) than low NS subjects, but this was not so clearly found using the NA scale where there were only significant differences for the pre-experimental condition ($F = 4.46$, df 1, 35, $P < 0.05$).

Tonic skin conductance

Thirty-six pre-stimulus measures of tonic skin conductance were estimated. In a 6-way analysis of variance with between-subjects factors of depressed patient/control, order (N-T/T-N), high/low Weinstein NS and within-subjects factors of noise/tone, intensity and repetitions there were significant main effects for noise/tone ($F = 7.1$, df 1, 28, $P < 0.02$) intensity ($F = 4.4$, df 2, 27, $P < 0.03$) and repetitions ($F = 2.9$, df 5, 24, $P < 0.04$). Tonic skin conductance was higher for all groups during exposure to noise rather than tone, except for high NS control subjects, who received noise first.

Tonic skin conductance levels were marginally higher for noises than tones across all three levels of intensity. There were highly significant three-way interactions between noise/tone, intensity and Weinstein NS ($F = 7.4$, df 2, 27, $P < 0.003$) and four-way interactions between noise/tone, intensity, order and sensitivity ($F = 11.3$, df 2, 27, $P < 0.0003$). There was a tendency for high NS groups to have higher tonic skin conductance than low NS groups except for the low NS control group which as it had only two subjects may be atypical. Unlike NS, tonic skin conductance tended to be lower for high NA rather than low NA groups.

Skin conductance response amplitude

Skin conductance response amplitude was examined in a six-way repeated measures analysis

of variance, with between-subjects factors of depressive/control, sensitivity high/low (NS and NA respectively) and order and, within-subjects factors of noise/tone, intensity, and repetitions. Response amplitude was first calculated as the difference between pre- and post-stimulus log skin conductance levels. NS, but not NA, demonstrated a small main effect of sensitivity ($F = 6.18$, df 1, 28, $P < 0.02$). There were two more substantial interactions between NS and intensity ($F = 8.0$, df 2, 27, $P < 0.002$) and NS and repetitions by intensity ($F = 3.9$, df 10, 19, $P < 0.006$) and a small effect of order by repetitions by intensity ($F = 3.4$, df 10, 19, $P < 0.02$). In Fig. 3 there is a tendency for habituation on the first four sounds followed by a short rise and fall in amplitude on the fifth and sixth sounds respectively. The pattern of habituation over the 6 repetitions is approximately similar in most groups except for 100 dBA for the high NS group where the amplitude begins to rise again after the fourth sound. High NS subjects both begin with larger amplitudes at all three intensities than low NS subjects and also take longer to habituate in terms of their response amplitude remaining larger at the sixth repetition (Fig. 3). This is strikingly the case for the high NS group exposed to 100 dBA. Thus, the hypothesis is partly confirmed that highly noise-

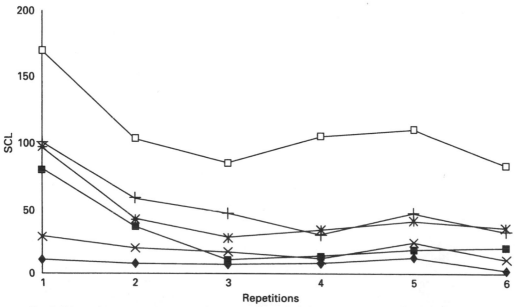

FIG. 3. Skin conductance response amplitude by sensitivity, intensity and repetitions. (□, High NS 100 dBA; +, low NS 100 dBA; ✳, high NS 75 dBA; ■, low NS 75 dBA; ×, high NS 50 dBA; ◆, low NS 50 dBA).

sensitive people are slower to habituate than low noise-sensitive people, but this occurs in relation to sound of high intensity rather than noise *versus* tone. The analyses were repeated using difference scores between post- and pre-stimulus skin conductance levels instead of log–log conductance levels. The same pattern of significant findings occurred for both NS and NA, except that the interactions between repetitions and noise/tone were lost and a small significant interaction was found between group by sensitivity and intensity by repetitions ($F = 3.3$, df 10, 19 $P < 0.02$).

Heart rate

Pre-stimulus heart rate was measured as interbeat interval for 5 s prior to each of the 36 stimuli. Data for each 5 s were averaged to provide one pre-stimulus value for each of the 36 stimuli. This was examined in a repeated measures analysis of variance with noise/tone, intensity and repetitions as within subject factors and depressive/control, sensitivity high or low, and order as between subject factors. There was a significant interaction between Weinstein NS and repetitions by Noise/Tone ($F = 3.4$, df 5, 24, $P < 0.02$) as well as an interaction between NS and noise/tone ($F = 5.6$, df 1, 28, $P < 0.03$). High NS subjects had faster heart rates than low

NS subjects for both noise and tone (Fig. 4). Tonic heart rate in high NS subjects rose across the six repetitions for exposure to noise and fell for exposure to tone. Among low NS subjects tonic heart rate fluctuated considerably but was little changed from the pre-experimental level after the 6 repetitions. For the NA analysis there was an interaction between noise/tone by intensity and NA ($F = 6.2$, df 2, 27, $P < 0.007$): as for the NS scale, high NA scorers had faster heart rates in both noise and tone conditions (Fig. 5). In addition, for high NA subjects heart rates were faster in noise than tone for all intensities, while for low NA subjects heart rate was faster in the noise condition than tone for 50 dBA, but was faster in the tone condition for 75 dBA and stayed virtually the same between noise and tone conditions for 100 dBA.

Heart rate responses

Heart rate was measured as interbeat interval for 10 s after the beginning of the stimulus. Each of the post-stimulus scores was subtracted from the mean pre-stimulus score to give 10 difference scores for each stimulus. These were analysed using repeated measures analysis of variance with between subjects factors of depressive/control, sensitivity (high/low), and order (N–T, T–N) and within subjects factors of noise/tone,

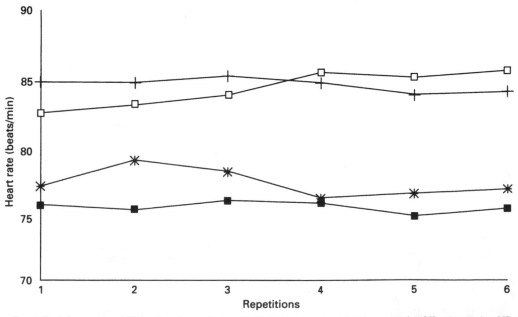

FIG. 4. Tonic heart rate and Weinstein noise sensitivity. (□, High NS noise; +, high NS tone; ✳, low NS noise; ■, low NS tone.)

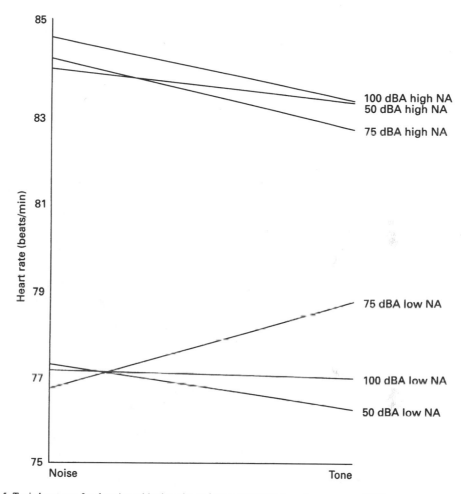

FIG. 5. Tonic heart rate for three intensities in noise and tone conditions for noise annoyance (NA) groups.

repetitions, intensity and magnitude. It was necessary to reduce the amount of data to make analysis more manageable. By reference to the previous literature (Turpin & Siddle, 1978) and observation of the raw data trends over the 10 time points, three 'windows' were defined. Immediately after the stimulus there was an initial deceleration. This was measured by the first 'window', between 1 and 2 s inclusively, where a single data point for each stimulus was the maximum amplitude value. The second 'window' between 3 and 5 s was designed to capture the accelerative response, and was comparable to Turpin and Siddle's (1978) work. In this 'window' the maximum accelerative value was taken for each stimulus. The final 'window' was between 6 and 9 s and captured

the 'late' decelerative response, the maximum amplitude response being used for each stimulus.

First 'window' (1–2 seconds post stimulus) In repeated measures analysis of variance there was a small significant interaction between NA and type of sound ($F = 4.95$, df 1, 28 $P < 0.04$) but this was not found for the Weinstein Scale.

Second window (3–5 seconds post stimulus) Repeated measures analysis of variance was employed with between-subjects factors of sensitivity, order, depression/control, and within subject factors of noise/tone, repetitions, intensity using the maximum accelerative value for each stimulus. There were significant main effects for type of sound in the NS analysis ($F = 12.06$,

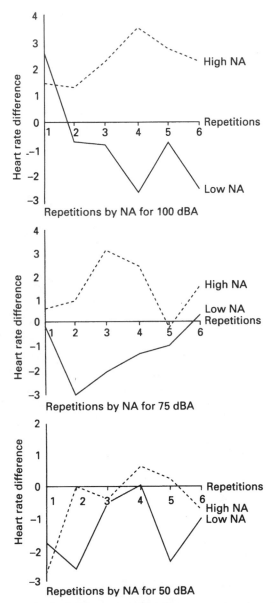

FIG. 6. Heart rate difference scores by noise annoyance, intensity and repetitions. (−−−, High noise annoyance; ——, low noise annoyance.)

df 1, 28, $P < 0.002$), in which there were greater accelerative responses to noises than to tones particularly for the first 6 sounds.

There were also significant interactions between noise/tone and repetitions ($F = 4.83$, df 5, 24, $P < 0.004$) where there were considerably greater accelerative responses to drill noise from the first 4 repetitions and noise/tone by repetitions by intensity ($F = 2.84$, df 10, 19, $P < 0.03$). When the maximum deflection was substituted for the maximum accelerative response there were significant main effects for NA ($F = 8.14$, df 1, 28, $P < 0.009$) and a significant interaction between NA and Noise/Tone by repetition by intensity ($F = 2.52$, df 10, 19, $P < 0.04$) but these were not found for the Weinstein Scale. For NA high scorers there were larger accelerative responses for both noise and tone and all three intensities than in NA lower scorers (Fig. 6). Also, high NA scorers tended to have more accelerative than decelerative responses across repetitions for 75 dBA and 100 dBA ($F = 2.16$, df 10, 19, $P < 0.08$).

Third 'window' (6–9 seconds) Repeated measures analysis of variance was used in a similar way to that for the first and second windows with the substitution of the value of maximum amplitude between 6 and 9 s. There were no significant main effects.

Discussion

The two studies reported here, following on from the previous study (Stansfeld *et al.* 1985 *a*, *b*), provide a model for investigating the associations of 'subjective' measures of noise sensitivity and psychiatric disorder while attempting to validate and complement these findings with 'objective' psychophysiological measurements. In the first study noise sensitivity was found to be a powerful predictor of noise annoyance and relatively stable over time. In the second study, noise sensitivity was associated with current psychiatric disorder and personality traits such as neuroticism. There was also some evidence for psychophysiological correlates of noise sensitivity in responsivity to noise. There was indirect evidence that noise sensitivity may be a risk factor for psychiatric disorder which is discussed below.

NOISE ANNOYANCE AND NOISE SENSITIVITY

A review of the literature on noise and psychiatric disorder demonstrates that environmental noise exposure leads to symptoms such as depression, tension, sleep disturbance and irritability but that these are limited to certain subgroups of the population and there is no evidence that noise alone is responsible for 'case-defined' psychiatric illness. Apart from noise level, subjective noise sensitivity has been found to be the most important predictor of the annoyance response (Taylor, 1984; Job, 1988). Aircraft noise specific annoyance has been related to both level of aircraft noise exposure and, independently, to noise sensitivity and psychiatric disorder (Tarnopolsky & Morton Williams, 1980). Despite this apparently central role, evidence from the West London survey does not suggest that annoyance is an intermediate step between noise and psychiatric disorder. Rather, it seems that both noise and pre-existing psychiatric disorder contribute to increasing annoyance. Noise sensitivity is a moderating variable explaining individual differences in annoyance. However, noise sensitivity is also associated with psychiatric disorder. Hence, the question of interest is whether noise sensitivity precedes psychiatric disorder and may be a risk factor for annoyance and psychiatric disorder, in particular, for psychiatric disorder caused by noise. Alternatively, is noise sensitivity secondary, a symptom of psychiatric disorder indistinguishable from annoyance?

A crucial question is how far noise sensitivity can be viewed as independent of annoyance. As has been indicated in the literature review the key distinction is that while annoyance is related to noise level, sensitivity is not. An indication of the role which noise sensitivity plays in annoyance is provided by Study 1, when being highly noise sensitive in 1977 both predicted higher and more consistent annoyance responses in 1980 and 1983 than being low sensitive in 1977. Again, in the previous community study (Stansfeld, 1989), when those with psychiatric disorder has been excluded, the further exclusion of those with low noise sensitivity increased the dependence of noise annoyance on noise level. Hence, there is evidence that noise sensitivity both determines and predicts the level of annoyance. It is clear though, in general, that noise sensitivity will mean high levels of annoyance for most noises, though not *all* noises, but more especially for those which the discriminating noise sensitive individual finds disturbing. For such disturbing noises the noise-sensitive individual remains highly consistently annoyed over long periods of time.

THE CONCEPT OF NOISE SENSITIVITY

If, as appears to be the case, noise sensitivity is not synonymous with annoyance, what is it? There is little evidence to suggest that noise sensitivity is entirely specific to noise. Evidence from the literature suggests moderately high correlations between noise sensitivity and sensitivity to other aspects of the environment. The general sensitivity measure used by Stansfeld *et al.* (1985 *a*) correlated moderately with noise sensitivity measures, although this correlation dropped substantially when 'possible cases' were excluded, suggesting that much of the common variance relates to morbidity factors.

STABILITY OF NOISE SENSITIVITY

If noise sensitivity is a predictor of annoyance, and may also be a predictor of minor psychiatric disorder, then surely a precondition must be that it remains stable to exert predictive power over a period of time. The results of previous studies of the reliability of noise sensitivity have been variable. In spite of the long interval and the methodological inadequacies of both the Self-Report and McKennell Scales of noise sensitivity in Study 1 there was a remarkable consistency across the two 3-year periods, with over 40% of the variance explained in the McKennell scale by the previous measure. This is in contrast to previous results with briefer measures (Griffiths & Delauzun, 1977) but in keeping with results using longer and more recent measures (Weinstein, 1978; Raw & Griffiths, 1988). Noise sensitivity was more consistent in high aircraft noise areas, perhaps because exposure to high noise levels tended to constantly remind people of their reactions to noise. The drift from low sensitivity to intermediate and high sensitivity over the three occasions is more difficult to explain. Certainly, while 'high' or 'more' noise sensitivity is relatively consistent over time, 'low' or 'less' sensitivity is inconsistent over time. It is possible that on recognizing the noise-related purpose of the study, subjects tended to respond more in the direction they expected they should to noise questions over time, but against this hypothesis there was little evidence from the EPQ (Eysenck & Eysenck, 1975) of a social desirability bias in noise sensitivity (see also Anderson, 1971) and much care was taken to disguise from subjects the primary interest in noise throughout the study.

It could be argued that because the original groups chosen for Study 1, were extreme groups on sensitivity they would be expected to remain more consistent on sensitivity than a general population sample. Thus, it was all the more striking that in Study 2, where changes in noise sensitivity were expected in conjunction with mood changes, both the Weinstein Scale and the NA scale of the Broadbent–Gregory General Annoyance Questionnaire demonstrated the same consistency across occasions four months apart in depressed patients as well as in matched control subjects. Nevertheless, four months may not be long enough to show much change attributable to recovery from depression.

On the whole, the evidence is strong for noise sensitivity being a stable trait with some consistency across different situations of noise exposure. However, noise sensitivity also implies discrimination in response to noise exposure (Weinstein, 1980) and discarding self-confessed variable individuals is not a solution, for, as Mischel (1968) has argued, variability is not synonymous with either capriciousness or unpredictability. Variability 'may well be the mark of a highly refined "discriminative facility", the ability to respond appropriately to subtle changes in situational contingencies' (Bem & Allen, 1974). Hence, some cross-situational inconsistency among highly noise sensitive people is not surprising. This is confirmed by the strong association between aircraft noise exposure (i.e. between two situations of high and low noise exposure) and annoyance found in Study 1 when low noise sensitive individuals are excluded (Stansfeld, 1989). Annoyance on the other hand is context dependent. For example, traffic noise heard out shopping is less annoying than traffic noise heard at home (Hedges, 1973). Nevertheless, there may be consistency in annoyance response even in imperturbable people, but because of less ability to discriminate rather than genuine indifference to noise and although adaptation to noise is known to be slow, people's opinions about noise often become fixed and remain so after only a few weeks' noise exposure (Weinstein, 1982).

In most people this propensity for being sensitive to noise lies dormant until the subject is exposed to noise (the provoking or eliciting context), when it is manifest as annoyance, a situation- and noise-specific response. Even within highly 'generally' noise-sensitive people there are likely to be certain noises which are more disturbing and others less so. Hence, if the greater discriminability of noise sensitive subjects is valid then annoyance will not always follow noise exposure. Nevertheless, Rushton et al. (1981) have found that the more extremely people rate their level on a personal trait, the more consistently do they rate themselves on that trait. Hence the more sensitive a person the more likely is he/she to be annoyed by a range of different noise sources. In summary, noise sensitive people may show greater variability in annoyance under different conditions of noise exposure than less sensitive people but will be more consistent in their annoyance responses over time.

NOISE SENSITIVITY AND PSYCHIATRIC DISORDER

If noise sensitivity indicates a subsample of the population vulnerable to the effects of noise there should be an association between noise sensitivity and psychiatric disorder. In the previous study (Stansfeld *et al.* 1985 *a*) between 40 % and 50 % of highly noise sensitive subjects were considered to be 'possible cases' of psychiatric disorder. While this indicates that a fairly large proportion of highly noise sensitive subjects are suffering from psychiatric symptoms, it does not mean that either the presence of psychiatric morbidity is a necessary prerequisite for reporting high sensitivity to noise or that noise sensitivity is merely a symptom of psychiatric morbidity.

In the scanty literature on noise sensitivity and psychiatric disorder there is a suggestion that noise sensitivity may be associated with severe depression, perhaps as a biological marker for low central serotoninergic activity, (Carman, 1973). This was not confirmed. Among depressed patients, ranging widely in severity and diagnosis, there was no evidence to support an association between noise sensitivity and major depression in particular, for mean noise sensitivity scores did not differ significantly between patients with psychotic, neurotic or retarded depressive illnesses classified by the PSE CATEGO program. As previously (Stansfeld *et al.* 1985 *a*), there was an association with the neurotic end of the spectrum of depressive illness. The higher PSE total symptom scores in highly noise sensitive patients were made up large of an excess of non-specific neurotic symptoms. There was no straightforward association between 'anxiety' symptoms and noise sensitivity; either with state or trait anxiety in the pilot study (Stansfeld, 1989) or with the anxiety subscale of the Symptom Rating Test, Nevertheless, high noise sensitivity on the McKennell Scale in Study 1 was significantly associated with the 'fear of aircraft noise' questions, suggesting an association with perception of threat even if not with overt anxiety.

It could be asked what evidence is to be found in Study 2 to confirm the association with psychiatric disorder found previously if it were not for the comparison between depressed patients and control subjects. Noise sensitivity scores were considerably higher in the depressed patients compared to the control subjects. High noise sensitivity is associated with a low level of psychiatric symptomatology, but one which is neither specifically 'depressive' nor 'anxious' in nature. The aspect of psychiatric morbidity with which it is associated seems to cut across, rather than be allied to, conventional diagnostic categories. In subjects where noise is related to phobic anxiety, it may be that noise sensitivity represents either specific noise phobia or is a marker for a general phobic tendency. Evidence for conditioned noise phobia is supported from studies of soldiers in war (Kipper, 1977), where severe and frequent anxiety reactions occurred in response to noises in some battle-exposed soldiers.

Noise sensitivity and recovery from depression

A way of testing whether noise sensitivity was secondary to depression was to examine noise sensitivity scores in relation to recovery from depression. Highly noise-sensitive subjects who made some recovery from depression between the two occasions of testing did become less sensitive (Study 2). This suggests that high noise sensitivity in these patients is partly secondary to current psychiatric state and that it diminishes as psychiatric symptoms lessen. Part of this drop in sensitivity scores, particularly in the highly noise sensitive group, is likely to be due to regression to the mean and is possibly an artefact of repeated testing. The useful internal comparison between noise sensitivity scores of those depressed patients who became worse and those who became better between the two occasions and the external comparison with the follow up of matched control subjects refutes the suggestion that this is all regression to the mean. Those who recovered from depression did become less noise sensitive, while those who became more depressed or remained unchanged also changed little in their noise sensitivity. The fall in the scores of the control subjects between the two occasions suggests an artefact of repeated testing but, nevertheless, the fall in sensitivity scores for depressed patients who recovered from depression is steeper than for their matched controls. It is interesting that even the noise sensitivity scores of the 'recovered' depressed patients are higher than their matched control subjects. This may mean that even between episodes of depression, depressed patients tend to have higher noise sensitivity scores than people who have never been depressed. One should be cautious about this conclusion because 'recovery' here is simply a drop in symptom rating test score between the two occasions, and although for this group there had been an improvement in clinical condition they were by no means fully recovered.

NOISE SENSITIVITY AND NEUROTICISM

If only part of the association between noise sensitivity and psychiatric disorder can be explained as noise sensitivity being secondary to illness, then is noise sensitivity more related to personality than current state? If this is the case then such personality measures may indicate special vulnerability to the effects of life stressors including noise. A consistent and significant association between noise sensitivity and neuroticism (range $r = 0.27 - 0.45$) was found in Studies 2 and previously (Stansfeld et al. 1985a). The size of the association is consistent with previous studies ($r = 0.36$, Anderson, 1971) ($r = 0.37$, Thomas & Jones, 1982). These findings and the association between noise sensitivity and asthenic subclinical symptoms (Stansfeld et al. 1985a) are echoed by Iwata's (1984) study of Japanese students where noise-sensitive individuals had more prominent symptoms of inadequacy, depression, anxiety, sensitivity, anger and tension on the Cornell Medical Index and more depression, inferiority and nervousness on the Yatabe–Guilford Personality Inventory. It seems likely that noise sensitivity is associated with a common pattern of morbidity identified by the non-specific neurotic symptoms of PSE, the inadequacy scale of the Symptom Rating Test, the neuroticism scale of the Eysenck

Personality Questionnaire and the asthenic subclinical symptoms which has been called negative affectivity (Watson & Clark, 1984).

According to the Foulds hierarchy model of psychiatric disorder (Foulds, 1965), this level of morbidity probably represents the bottom layer of the pyramid. This renders it no less important, for what it lacks in severity is made up for by the number of people affected. It is likely to contain symptoms related to fatigue, anergia, poor concentration, somatic symptoms such as headaches and sleep difficulties. This level of morbidity is particularly significant because it occupies a borderland between overt clinical psychiatric disorder and neurotic aspects of the personality and may indicate steps on the pathway to overt psychiatric disorder. When current psychiatric disorder and neuroticism are measured on the same occasion, as in Study 2 among depressed patients, there is always a possibility that current disorder will contaminate measures of neuroticism. That the association between noise sensitivity and neuroticism is not merely an artefact of an association with psychiatric disorder is shown by an association between noise sensitivity and neuroticism of similar magnitude with the control subjects in Study 2 who, by definition and confirmed by Symptom Rating Test (SRT) scores, were not suffering from current psychiatric disorder.

This result suggests that noise sensitivity, already demonstrated to be a fairly stable trait, is associated with a cluster of personal characteristics and subclinical symptoms of neuroticism/negative affectivity, in the absence of frank psychiatric morbidity, but which may predict the future appearance of psychiatric morbidity provoked by other agents. However, Study 1 was not a sufficient test of noise sensitivity as a predictor of psychiatric morbidity.

The borderline between psychiatric morbidity and neuroticism is somewhat artificial and both may represent measures of an underlying stable level of psychiatric symptomatology (Duncan Jones et al. 1990). But because neuroticism tends to be present over a longer period of time than overt clinical psychiatric morbidity does not mean that neuroticism is a fixed state. It may be that neuroticism represents, in certain cases, the mild but longer-term precursor or postscript of overt illness, or represents a temporary period of subclinical 'illness' with possibilities for 're-covery' and a life without neuroticism.

There is a danger in getting immersed in the associations between noise sensitivity, neuroti-cism and psychiatric disorder where the bound-aries between psychiatric disorder and neur-oticism are evanescent and the directions of association ultimately uncertain. Such a 'slough of despond' may reasonably be left behind in the search for a biological correlate for noise sensitivity. This might act as an 'objective' index of psychiatric vulnerability uncontaminated by response bias.

NOISE SENSITIVITY AND HEARING THRESHOLD

In attempting both to validate noise sensitivity and to search for evidence of psycho-physiological vulnerability to stressors ac-companying noise sensitivity it seemed important to search for associations with likely biological parameters which were not measured by ques-tionnaires and which might be free of the response bias which self-report questionnaires inevitably entail. First, it was important to exclude any association between noise sensitivity and hearing threshold measured by audiometry. There was no such association either in Study 2 or previously (Stansfeld *et al.* 1985*b*). Excluding the few persons with gross hearing loss seems unlikely to have compromised a possible as-sociation. This lack of association is not surprising: the level of absolute hearing thresh-old does not necessarily determine the response of the ear to suprathreshold sounds; in par-ticular, having lower hearing thresholds does not necessarily mean that suprathreshold sounds would be perceived as louder by these persons.

Is noise sensitivity synonymous with hyper-acusis or phonophobia? Phonophobia, or in-tolerance of loud noise, is the commonest symptomatic accompaniment of migrainous headache (Kayan & Hood, 1984). Phonophobia is a time-limited state response which may contribute to a person's perception of being generally sensitive to noise but is not the same as noise sensitivity measured by questionnaire. Kayan & Hood (1984) suggest that loudness recruitment causes phonophobia, resulting from transient disturbance of cochlear receptor func-tion, consequent upon arterial vasoconstriction.

If so, might this mechanism contribute to noise sensitivity in general? Noise sensitivity has been related to peripheral vasoconstriction (Cohen *et al.* 1973) and it may be that part of the common variance shared between noise sen-sitivity and neuroticism is explained by auto-nomic instability, proneness to episodic cerebral vasoconstriction and hence loudness recruit-ment. In addition, noise sensitivity is sometimes associated with hearing impairment (Gordon, 1986; Aniansson *et al.* 1983) and noise induced hearing loss and with poor cochlear frequency selectivity (Najenson *et al.* 1988). Noise-sensitive listeners also perform less well on speech tests in the presence of white-noise masking, suggesting signal-to-noise perceptual deficit which requires further investigation (Abel *et al.* 1988).

PSYCHOPHYSIOLOGICAL CORRELATES OF NOISE SENSITIVITY

In most people psychophysiological responses to noise, in terms of heart rate and skin conductance, rapidly habituate unless the noise source has some potent meaning such as an indicator of threat. A small minority of people do not habituate to noise or only habituate very slowly. Are these people noise sensitive, aware of their own physiological sensitivity to noise and hence score highly on self-report ques-tionnaires? One should be cautious in linking psychophysiological results to subjective meas-ures; the methodological problems in psycho-physiological measurement are formidable, the correlations between mood and measures such as heart rate are modest (Morrow & Labrum, 1978; Johnston & Anastasiades, 1990) and inconsistent, even in normal subjects (Turner *et al.* 1990) and experimental demand charac-teristics may be powerful and undetected by the experimenter. Do high noise-sensitive subjects have high levels of physiological arousal? Van Dijk (1986) has suggested that their level of arousal may have an important effect on coping with noise, and studies of performance have found arousal to be an important moderating variable (Broadbent, 1983).

Tonic skin conductance and heart rate

The initial investigation of psychophysiological measurements in extreme groups of noise-sensitive women performed in the community was a radical step forward in attempting to get ecological validity for psychophysiological measurement in response to environmental noise. However, there were major difficulties in controlling the non-noise aspects of the environment which might influence heart rate and skin conductance. Hence it was felt appropriate, once more, to look for differences in responsivity to noise among noise sensitive subjects in the laboratory. Ideally, it would have been better to have chosen extreme groups of noise sensitivity for the laboratory experiment, but in practice this was not possible. In study 2, high noise-sensitive subjects did seem to have higher levels of arousal than low noise-sensitive subjects in terms of more spontaneous fluctuations (Hart, 1974) both pre- and post-experimentally and higher tonic skin conductance level, and faster tonic heart rates for both noise and tone. This is in keeping with studies of patients with chronic anxiety states (Bond et al. 1974), but not depressed patients. As far as tonic skin conductance is concerned, noise-sensitive subjects seem more like those with anxiety than depression and the laboratory findings are in accordance with noise sensitivity being related to high arousal. Moreover, for high NS subjects exposed to noise, tonic heart rate rose across the experiment, while it fell for exposure to tones. This suggests that high noise sensitive subjects became more aroused by continuous noxious noise but gradually less aroused by continuous less noxious tones. This favours greater discrimination of response to sound in noise sensitive subjects. The apparent discrepancy between the results in the previous study (Stansfeld et al. 1985b) where tonic heart rates were lower in sensitive subjects, and Study 2 where they were higher, may relate to context. In the previous study heart rates were not related to noise stimuli, while in the laboratory study tonic heart rates were measured in the context of attention to further noise stimuli.

Phasic skin conductance and heart rate responses

Skin conductance response amplitude was larger for both noises *versus* tones and increased with increasing intensity. In line with this finding high NS, but not high NA, subjects tended initially to have larger skin conductance response amplitudes. This is not similar to the findings in anxious patients where Lader & Wing (1966) and Hart (1974) found similar higher levels of tonic skin conductance, but smaller responses to initial stimulation or differences between anxious and control subjects. The findings with noise sensitivity are, however, similar to those found by Öhman et al. (1974) in normal subjects exposed to potentially phobic stimuli where skin conductance responses to a phobic visual stimulus were significantly larger than to a neutral visual stimulus. This physiological response in noise-sensitive subjects may indicate fear of noise stimuli. For phasic heart rate response difference scores, examined as maximum deflection (i.e. amplitude rather than magnitude; Turpin & Siddle, 1978), in the second window (3–5 s post-stimulus: Turpin & Siddle 1983), high NA scorers had larger accelerative responses to noise and tone than low NA scorers across all three intensities, and for 75 dBA and 100 dBA in particular they tended to maintain an accelerative response across repetitions, suggesting slower habituation of defence/startle reactions to more intense noises in noise sensitive subjects. This must be considered a preliminary finding because it was not statistically significant when only accelerative responses were considered and it was also not significant for the Weinstein scale, although a similar pattern exists in the mean scores. Turpin & Siddle (1983) found a similar pattern of accelerative response to high intensities of sound but no differences in habituation between accelerative and decelerative components. Thus, although these findings are not wholly consistent, there is a suggestion that noise sensitivity is associated with higher levels of physiological arousal to noise, phobic and defence/startle responses to noise and slower habituation to noise. Such physiological findings may be related to the greater annoyance responses in noise sensitive subjects and form the basis for a mechanism for stressor induced health effects.

FACTORS UNDERLYING NOISE SENSITIVITY

In summary, from these studies, it seems that noise sensitivity does predict annoyance and is related to both current psychiatric disorder and neuroticism. It has not been proved that noise sensitivity predicts later psychiatric disorder. Indeed, part of noise sensitivity is secondary to depressive illness but it seems in these persons it is usually superimposed on already high levels of trait sensitivity. Nevertheless, noise sensitivity is relatively stable across time and is related to slower habituation of heart rate responses to loud threatening noises.

Perceptions of threat and control and noise sensitivity

Why should sensitivity to noise be associated with predisposition to psychiatric disorder? Sensitivity to noise is probably not a vulnerability factor for psychiatric disorder caused specifically by noise exposure. It seems more likely that noise sensitivity is a self-perceived indicator of vulnerability to stressors in general. Noise sensitive people might perceive more threat from external events than other people. This might either be because of greater awareness of external events (Weinstein's critical tendencies) or because they interpret these events as more threatening (locus of control, Thomas & Jones, 1982). As well as attentional factors, higher levels of physiological arousal may contribute to this greater awareness of external events. This perception of greater threat is backed up by the phobic responses to noise on skin conductance and the slower habituation of the defence/startle response on heart rate in noise-sensitive subjects in the laboratory experiment. Fraser (1932) has commented that primitive man relied upon his hearing more than modern man, and the emotion of fear is still the first idea which arises in association with any strange noise. Thus hearing is a primary sense for the appreciation of threat and, by invoking Seligman's concept of 'belongingess' (McNally, 1987), strange noises might be readily perceived as threatening by those who are so predisposed. It may be hypothesized that some people are 'biologically prepared' (McNally, 1987) to associate certain noises with threat but that this preparedness either varies within different people (Öhman *et al.* 1985) or the range of noises involved varies across different people. According to this formulation, noise-sensitive people would be those most 'biologically prepared' for noise. The perception of threat might also occur

because the subjects may perceive external stressors, such as noise, to be either unpredictable or uncontrollable or both, and a perception of non-contingency may lead to learned helplessness (Burger & Arkin, 1980). Additionally, it may be that perception of external threat is a result of projection of feelings of hostility on to the external world and indicates a paranoid mechanism.

Negative affectivity and greater reactions to noise

On the other hand, perception may be unexceptional but nevertheless individuals may tend to react more readily or more strongly to possible external threat (e.g. Philips & Hunter's (1982) migraine subjects). Again this is supported by the higher levels of arousal in noise sensitive subjects in the laboratory experiment. This is reminiscent of Taylor's (1984) distinction between sensitivity and annoyance. It is clear that only some noise sensitive people express annoyance when they are exposed to noise. This suggests that other factors moderate the annoyance response to noise in sensitive individuals. One such factor might be described as a general tendency to be angry or at least to report annoyance. This might also explain the consistency of noise annoyance over time. But what is this general tendency to anger? It may be related to 'plaintive set', that is a tendency to report things more negatively, especially on self-report questionnaires. Henderson (1981) quotes Gruenberg's term as 'a propensity for complaining and being generally dissatisfied with a wide range of elements in day-to-day living'. 'Plaintive set' is not the same as active complaint behaviour related to noise, which requires more active behaviour than merely voicing the complaint. It might thus be easy to dismiss noise sensitivity as merely 'response bias' but underlying 'plaintive set' may be negative affectivity (Watson & Clark, 1984); a 'mood-dispositional' dimension of negative emotionality (including nervousness, anger, and dissatisfaction) and negative self concept. This could be seen as largely independent of any specific provoking agent. This is supported by evidence that sensitive individuals react affectively to noise while non-sensitive individuals react cognitively to noise (Finke *et al.* 1974). It is interesting that although negative affectivity is very similar to noise sensitivity it does not seem to relate to a general phobic tendency which noise sensitivity does (Watson & Clark, 1984). It seems likely that noise sensitivity is made up of these two elements. The perception of greater threat and less control over the environment can be combined with the tendency to negative affectivity. It seems likely that excessive sensitivity to environmental stimuli would be preceded by a previously learned or biologically prepared attribution of greater threat from stimuli, hence greater awareness of threat would lead to a lower threshold of reactivity. Noise sensitive people may attend more readily to noises, perceive more threat from noises and react more readily both psychologically and physically to noises than people who are not sensitive.

In this case noise would act as a stimulus with implications of threat but would have little direct effect related to the physical parameters of the sound (Tarnopolsky *et al.* 1980). However, in real life, environmental noise exposure is unlikely to rank very highly among the many other threatening environmental stressors to which people are exposed.

Nevertheless, noise might have some direct effect on health when a person is aware of their less than resilient reaction to previous stressors or when, under pressure from current stressors, they are at the limits of their coping capacity then they may tend to perceive noise as an additional and tiresome stressor. It has been suggested (Eysenck, 1982) that arousal and anxiety lead to a narrowing of attention to external stimuli because of preoccupation with internal stimuli. In this context external noise may be a distracting influence which puts excessive strain on a failing attentional mechanism in an anxious person. Prolonged exposure to situations inducing learned helplessness such as admission to hospital (Raps *et al.* 1982) has been shown to increase vulnerability to performance deficits caused by noise. Thus noise may be having a greater effect on the already impaired individual. This may be particularly so in people suffering from overt or subclinical psychiatric disorder where their usual capacity for coping is restricted. An extreme version of helplessness is displayed by the Intensive Care Unit patient, immobilized by severe illness, possibly in pain, and sleep deprived and exposed

to a range of incomprehensible and threatening noises; in this situation sensitivity to noise and subsequent disturbance is often reported and is considered a contribution to 'ICU psychosis' (Hansell, 1984).

Another setting of exposure to multiple stressors is the battlefield where conditioning to noise phobias in battle-exposed soldiers is instructive (Kipper, 1977). Noise phobias have been reported in settings where there was a realization of extreme danger, with perceived inability to cope effectively with threat and often in conditions of mental or physical fatigue. Their occurrence was subsequently associated with a general deterioration in coping and negative self-evaluation. The question then arises of whether greater perceived threat from environmental stimuli in patients with minor psychiatric morbidity is primary, or secondary, to disorder. If it is secondary then it might be explained in terms of the halo effect of depressed mood, when everything in the depressed patients' world, both external and internal, is interpreted as gloomy and negative or as threatening, as a result of the patient's primary disturbance of mood. On the other hand, it might be that increased perception of threat in noise-sensitive individuals precedes, and is a risk factor for, the development of psychiatric disorder. Although the psychophysiological results suggest an 'objective' biological correlate of increased threat in noise-sensitive patients, which is independent of any effect of depression, a longitudinal study would be needed to be certain that this preceded depression.

In summary, noise sensitivity may be comprised of two elements. Noise is important to noise-sensitive people who attend to noises more, discriminate between noises more, and tend to find noises more threatening and out of their control than people who are not sensitive to noise. Secondly, because of negative affectivity, they react to noises more than less sensitive people, and may adapt to noises more slowly. This may result in a greater expression of annoyance to noises than in less sensitive people, both because this a response to greater threat and also because they may have a general tendency to be annoyed, irrespective of noise. Both these latter factors may be active in explaining the association between noise sensitivity and current psychiatric disorder and explaining why noise sensitivity is a vulnerability factor for psychiatric disorder.

Environmental noise does not cause clinically defined psychiatric disorder in the population but it does lead to psychological symptoms in certain subgroups of the population. This means that there is a differential vulnerability to the effects of noise within the population which may apply to the environmental stressors as a whole.

Noise as an example of an environmental stressor may serve as an analogy for the pathogenic effects of other environmental stressors. Such stressors, defined in the broadest sense, would include those classified in the sociomedical literature as life events and chronic difficulties. The meaning of the noise for the individual is the central feature of such vulnerability to noise effects, typified by noise sensitivity. Within this concept, the perception of increased threat from noise, the belief of lack of control over noise, the increased physiological reactivity, the slower adaptation to noise and pre-existing negative affectivity are the component perceptions, attitudes and reactions which indicate that some people develop psychological symptoms while others do not.

THE NEED FOR FURTHER RESEARCH

First, there is a need for methodological refinement in the measurement of both annoyance and noise sensitivity. Noise annoyance measurements would be much strengthened by unobtrusive measures of behaviour, by measures comparing annoyance levels to easily comprehensible standard levels of annoyance and by measures which take greater account of context. Improvements in the reliability, simplicity and comprehensiveness of noise sensitivity measurement would be welcome.

Secondly, there needs to be greater sophistication in research design which will allow comparison between annoyance measures, sensitivity measures and standardized instruments measuring other psychological states such as anger, response patterns such as negative affectivity, behaviours such as aggression, varied health endpoints, and passive and active coping methods. Ideally, such research should be carried out in a setting of meaningful noise with due attention to contextual factors in terms of socioeconomic position, social networks, culture, and

other environmental stimulation. In particular, there needs to be further research to tease apart the subcomponents of noise sensitivity. This has particular relevance to the understanding of the association with minor psychiatric disorder. The question of which subcomponents of noise sensitivity (increased threat perception, negative affectivity, perceived vulnerability, greater affective reactivity) are merely secondary to psychiatric morbidity has not been clearly established. If measurable increased perception of threat from environmental stressors were to precede minor psychiatric disorder in the causal chain, this would have profound implications for work on the prevention of minor psychiatric disorder. This would link with the work on locus of control and self efficacy important as determinants of health in other contexts (Syme, 1991).

Future work needs to examine these subcomponents in a general population sample in order to tease out the temporal sequence of these changes in the evolution of minor psychiatric disorder. It is simplistic, if operationally convenient, to separate these factors as being either primary or secondary to disorder. This ignores the decision about when a subclinical disorder becomes a clinical illness, and it blurs the fact that once a borderline illness is established these factors may continue to exert a pathological effect through feedback mechanisms. Of particular importance in this respect is the effect of community noise exposure on those people who have either subclinical or established minor psychiatric disorder. Can noise in these people lead to a worsening of their condition?

In a wider context the debate still continues: does noise cause psychiatric disorder? The meticulous West London study does not seem to have been accepted as the final word for several reasons, partly to do with its method. A cross-sectional study, however carefully carried out, cannot be expected to answer questions of causation. The lack of association between noise exposure and psychiatric morbidity found cross-sectionally does rule out any large effect of noise, but this study is potentially flawed by problems of selection of people into different noise exposure areas before the study was carried out. There is a suggestion that those who lived in the high noise area were noise 'survivors', those who are intolerant of noise, particularly in the greater than 55 NNI area, having already moved out. For the 'survivors' the incentives to remain or to move into the area are related to lower property prices. The problem with the low noise areas is that they were not as homogeneous in social class as the high-noise areas. Some low-noise areas were wealthier and healthier, other areas poorer and contained an excess of ill health which might have obscured any small effect due to noise. To determine whether noise contributes to the development of psychiatric disorder a prospective study is needed in which a cohort is examined at baseline period, exposed to environmental noise over time, and the development of psychiatric disorder observed. Ideally, this should take place in a population where the initial noise exposure is low and thus the population selection factors are absent. Such studies should incorporate the methodological refinements mentioned and, with the aid of a more comprehensive model of noise annoyance and noise sensitivity, examine the complex interplay of their subcomponents in the pathways to ill health.

REFERENCES

Abel, S. M., Alberti, P. W. & Krever, E. M. (1988). Auditory function and speech perception in noise in aging and noise sensitive listeners. *Noise 88. Noise as a Public Health Problem. Vol 2: Hearing, communication, sleep and non-auditory physiological effects* (ed. B. Berglund), pp. 223–227. Swedish Council for Building Research: Stockholm.

Abey-Wickrama, I., A'Brook, M. F., Gattoni, F. E. G. & Herridge, C. F. (1969). Mental hospital admissions and aircraft noise. *Lancet* **633**, 1275–1277.

Anderson, C. M. B. (1971). *The Measurement of Attitude to Noise and Noises. National Physical Laboratory Acoustics report, Ac 52.* Teddington, Middx.

Aniansson, G., Pettersson, R. & Peterson, Y. (1983). Traffic noise annoyance and noise sensitivity in persons with normal and impaired hearing. *Journal of Sound and Vibration* **88**, 85–96.

Arguelles, A. E. (1967). Endocrine response to auditory stress of normal and psychotic subjects. In *Endocrinology and Human Behavior* (ed. R. P. Michael), p. 200. Oxford University Press: New York.

Arguelles, A. E., Martinez, M. A., Pucciarelli, E. & Disisto, M. V. (1970). Endocrine and metabolic effects of noise in normal, hypertensive and psychotic subjects. In *Physiological Effects of Noise* (ed. B. Welch), pp. 43–55. Plenum Press: New York.

Atherley, G. R. C., Gibbons, S. L. & Powell, J. A. (1970). Moderate acoustic stimuli: the interrelation of subjective importance and certain physiological changes. *Ergonomics* **13**, 536–545.

Babisch, W., Ising, H., Gallacher, J. E. J. & Elwood, P. C. (1988). Traffic noise and cardiovascular risk. The Caerphilly study, first phase. Outdoor noise levels and risk factors. *Archives of Environmental Health* **43**, 407–414.

Barbenza, C. M., McRoberts, M. & Tempest, W. (1970). Individual loudness functions. *Journal of Sound and Vibration* **11**, 399–410.

Barker, S. M. & Tarnopolsky, A. (1978). Assessing bias in surveys of symptoms attributed to noise. *Journal of Sound & Vibration* **59**, 349–354.

Beardwood, C. J. (1982). Hormonal changes associated with auditory stimulation. In *Handbook of Psychiatry and Endocrinology* (ed. P. J. V. Beumont and G. D. Burrows), pp. 401–441. Elsevier Biomedical Press: Amsterdam.

Bem, D. J., Allen, A. (1974). On predicting some of the people some of the time: the search for cross-situational consistencies in behaviour. *Psychological Review* **81**, 506–520.

Bennett, E. (1945). Some tests for the discrimination of neurotic from normal subjects. *British Journal of Medical Psychology* **20**, 271–277.

Berglund, B., Berglund, U. & Lindvall, T. (1976). Scaling loudness, noisiness and annoyance of community noises. *Journal of the Acoustic Society of America* **60**, 119–125.

Bond, A. J., James, C. D. & Lader, M. H. (1974). Physiological and psychological measures in anxious patients. *Psychological Medicine* **4**, 364–373.

Borsky, P. N. (1961). *Community Reactions to Air Force Noise. I. Basic Concepts and Preliminary Methodology. II. Data on Community Studies and their Interpretation.* Rept. TR 60-689, Contract A.F. 41 (657)-79. National Opinion Research Center, University of Chicago.

Borsky, P. N. (1980). *Review of Community Response to Noise. Proceedings IIIrd International Congress on Noise as a Public Health Problem.* ASHA Reports Number 10: Rockville, USA.

Bowsher, J. M., Johnson, D. R. & Robinson, D. W. (1966). A further experiment on judging the noisiness of aircraft in flight. *Acustica* **17**, 245–267.

Bregman, H. L. & Pearson, R. G. (1972). *Development of a Noise Annoyance Sensitivity Scale.* National Aeronautics and Space Administration CR-1954 National Technical Information Service: Springfield, Virginia 22151.

Broadbent, D. E. (1953). Noise, paced performance, and vigilance tasks. *British Journal of Psychology* **44**, 295–303.

Broadbent, D. E. (1972). Individual differences in annoyance by noise. *Sound* **6**, 56–61.

Broadbent, D. E. (1983). Recent advances in understanding performance in noise. *Proceedings of Fourth International Congress, Noise as a Public Health Problem.* Volume 2 (ed. G. Rossi), pp. 719–738. Centro Ricerche e studi amplifon: Milano.

Broadbent, D. E., Cooper, P. F., Fitzgerald, P. & Parkes, K. R. (1982). The Cognitive Failures Questionnaire (CFQ) and its correlates. *British Journal of Clinical Psychology* **21**, 1–16.

Bugard, P., Souvras, H., Valade, P., Coste, E. & Salle, J. (1953). Le Syndrome de fatigue et les troubles auditifs des metteurs au point d'aviation. *La Semaine des Hopitaux* **29**, 65–70.

Bullen, R. B., Hede A. J. & Kyriacos, E. (1986). Reaction to aircraft noise in residential areas around Australian airports. *Journal of Sound and Vibration* **108**, 199–225.

Burger, J. M. & Arkin, R. M. (1980). Prediction, control and learned helplessness. *Journal of Personality and Social Psychology* **38**, 482–491.

Burns, W. (1973). *Noise and Man.* John Murray: London.

Cameron, P., Robertson, D. & Zaks, J. (1972). Sound pollution, noise pollution and health: community parameters. *Journal of Applied Psychology* **56**, 67–74.

Carman, J. S. (1973). Imipramine in hyperacusic depression. *American Journal of Psychiatry* **130**, 937.

Chowns, R. H. (1970). Mental hospital admissions and aircraft noise. *Lancet* i, 467–468.

Civil Aviation Authority. (1980). *Aircraft Noise and Sleep Disturbance: Final Report.* DORA Report 8008: London.

Cohen, H. H., Conrad, D. W., O'Brien, J. F. & Pearson, R. G. (1973). Noise effects, arousal and human processing task difficulty and performance. *Human Factors* March 1973, North Carolina State University at Raleigh.

Cohen, A. (1976). The influence of a company hearing conservation program on extra-auditory problems in workmen. *Journal of Public Safety* **8**, 146–161.

Cohen, S., Evans, G. W., Krantz, D. S., Stokols, D. (1980). Physiological, motivational and cognitive effects of aircraft noise on children. *American Psychologist* **35**, 231–243.

Cohen, S. & Spacapan, S. (1978). The after effects of stress: an attentional interpretation. *Environmental Psychology and Nonverbal Behavior* **3**, 43–57.

Cohen, S. & Weinstein, N. (1981). Non-auditory effects of noise on behaviour and health. *Journal of Social Issues* **37**, 36–70.

Cooper, A. F., Curry, A. R., Kay, D. W. K., Garside, R. F. & Roth, M. (1974). Hearing loss and affective psychoses of the elderly. *Lancet* ii, 851–854.

Crook, M. A. & Langdon, F. J. (1974). The effects of aircraft noise in schools around London Airport. *Journal of Sound and Vibration* **34**, 221–232.

Davies, D. R. & Hockey, G. R. J. (1966). The effects of noise and doubling the signal frequency on individual differences in visual vigilance performance. *British Journal of Psychology* **57**, 381–389.

Davis, H. (1958). (ed.) *Project Anehin USN School of Aviation Medicine,* Project NM 130199, Subtask 1, Report No. 7: Pensacola, Florida.

Di Nisi, J., Muzet, A. & Weber, L. D. (1987). Cardiovascular responses to noise effects of self-estimated sensitivity to noise, sex, and time of day. *Journal of Sound and Vibration* **114**, 271–279.

Duncan-Jones, P., Fergusson, D. M., Ormel, J. & Horwood, L. J. (1990). *A Model of Stability and Change in Minor Psychiatric*

Symptoms: Results from Three Longitudinal Studies. Psychological Medicine Monograph Supplement 18. Cambridge University Press: Cambridge.

Evans, G. W. & Tafalla, R. (1987). Measurement of environmental annoyance. In Developments in Toxicology and Environmental Science (ed. H. S. Koelaga), pp. 11–25. Elsevier: Amsterdam.

Eysenck, H. J. & Eysenck, S. B. G. (1975). Manual of the Eysenck Personality Questionnaire. Hodder and Stoughton: London.

Eysenck, M. W. (1982). Attention and Arousal. Springer Verlag: Berlin.

Fields, J. M. (1984). The effect of numbers of noise events on people's reactions to noise. An analysis of existing survey data. Journal of the Acoustic Society of America 75, 447–467.

Finke, H. O., Guski, R., Martin, R., Rohrmann, B., Schümer, R. & Schümer-Kohrs, A. (1974). Effects of aircraft noise on man. Proceedings of the Symposium on Noise in Transportation, section III, paper 1. Institute of Sound and Vibration Research: Southampton.

Fog, H. & Jonsson, E. (1968). Traffic Noise in Residential Areas. Report 36E, National Swedish Institute for Building Research: Stockholm.

Foulds, G. A. (1965). Personality and Personal Illness. Tavistock, London.

Fraser, D. (1932). The psychological effects of noise. Medical Journal of Australia 1, 50.

Frerichs, R. R., Beeman, B. L. & Coulson, A. H. (1980). Los Angeles Airport noise and mortality – faulty analysis and public policy. American Journal of Public Health 70, 357–362.

Fuller, H. C. & Robinson, D. W. (1973). Subjective Reactions to Steady and Varying Noise Environments. NPL Acoustics Report. AC 62: Teddington, Middlesex.

Gang, M. J. & Teft, L. (1975). Individual differences in heart rate responses to affective sound. Psychophysiology 12, 423–426.

Gattoni, F. & Tarnopolsky, A. (1973). Aircraft noise and psychiatric morbidity. Psychological Medicine 3, 516–520.

Glass, D. C. & Singer, J. E. (1972). Urban Stress. Academic Press: New York.

Globus, G., Friedmann, J., Cohen, H., Pearsons, K. S. & Fidell, S. (1973). The effects of aircraft noise on sleep electrophysiology as recorded in the home. Proceedings of the International Congress on Noise as a Public Health Problem (ed. Ward, W. D.), pp. 587–592. US Environmental Protection Agency: Washington, DC.

Goldberg, D. P. (1972). The Detection of Psychiatric Illness by Questionnaire. Oxford University Press: London.

Goldberg, D. P., Cooper, B., Eastwood, M. R., Kedward, H. B. & Shepherd, M. (1970). A standardized psychiatric interview suitable for use in community surveys. British Journal of Preventive and Social Medicine 24, 18–23.

Gordon, A. G. (1986). Abnormal middle ear muscle reflexes and audiosensitivity. British Journal of Audiology 20, 95–99.

Granati, A., Angelepi, F. & Lenzi, R. (1959). L'influenza dei rumori sul sistema nervoso. Folia Medica 42, 1313–1325.

Graeven, D. B. (1975). Necessity, control and predictability of noise as determinants of noise annoyance. Journal of Social Psychology 95, 85–90.

Grandjean, E., Graf, P., Cauber, A., Meier, H. P. and Muller, R. (1973). A survey of aircraft noise in Switzerland. Proceedings of the International Congress on Noise as a Public Health Problem, Dubrovnik, pp. 645–659. US Environmental Protection Agency Publications, 500/973-008: Washington, DC.

Griffiths, I. D. & Delauzun, F. R. (1977). Individual differences in sensitivity to traffic noise: an empirical study. Journal of Sound and Vibration 55, 93–107.

Griffiths, I. D. & Langdon, F. J. (1968). Subjective Response to road traffic noise. Journal of Sound and Vibration 8, 16–32.

Gulian, E. (1974). Noise as an Occupational Hazard: Effects of Performance Level. National Institute of Occupational Safety and Health: Cincinnati, Ohio.

Gunn, W. J. (1987). The importance of the measurement of annoyance in prediction of effects of aircraft noise on the health and well-being of noise exposed communities. In Developments in

Toxicology and Environmental Science (ed. H. S. Koelaga), pp. 237–255. Elsevier: Amsterdam.

Gunn, W. J., Shigehisa, T., Fletcher, J. L. & Shepherd, W. T. (1981). Annoyance response to aircraft noise as a function of contextual effects and personality characteristics. Journal of Auditory Research 21, 51–83.

Hall, F. L., Taylor, S. M. & Birnie, S. E. (1985). Activity interference and noise annoyance. Journal of Sound and Vibration 103, 237–252.

Hamilton, M. (1967). Development of a rating scale for primary depressive illness. British Journal of Social and Clinical Psychology 6, 278–296.

Hansell, H. N. (1984). The behavioral effects of noise on man: the patient with 'intensive care unit psychosis'. Heart and Lung 13, 59–65.

Hart, J. O. (1974). Physiological responses of anxious and normal subjects to simple signal and non-signal auditory stimuli. Psychophysiology 11, 443–451.

Hazard, W. R. (1971). Predictions of noise disturbance near large airports. Journal of Sound and Vibration 15, 425–445.

Hedges, B. (1973). Road Traffic and the Environment – Preliminary Report. Social and Community Planning Research: 35 Northampton Square, London, E.C.1.

Henderson, A. S. (1981). Neurosis and the Social Environment. Academic Press: Sydney.

Hockey, G. R. J. (1970). Effect of loud noise on attentional selectivity. Quarterly Journal of Experimental Psychology 22, 28–36.

Ising, H., Dienel, D., Günther, T. & Market, B. (1980). Health effects of traffic noise. International Archives of Occupational and Environmental Health 47, 179–190.

Ising, H., Rebentisch, E., Poustka, F. & Cuiro, I. (1990). Annoyance and health risk by military low-altitude flight noise. International Archives of Occupational and Environmental Health 62, 357–363.

Iwata, O. (1984). The relationship of noise sensitivity to health and personality. Japanese Psychological Research 26, 75–81.

Jansen, G. (1961). Adverse effects of noise in iron and steel workers. Stahl und Eisen 81, 217–220.

Jansen, G. (1969). Effects of noise on physiological state. American Speech and Hearing Association Reports, no. 4, 89–98.

Jenkins, L. M., Tarnopolsky, A., Hand, D. J., Barker, S. M. (1979). Comparison of three studies of aircraft noise and psychiatric hospital admissions conducted in the same area. Psychological Medicine 9, 681–693.

Jenkins, L. M., Tarnopolsky, A. & Hand, D. J. (1981). Psychiatric admissions and aircraft noise from London Airport: four-year, three hospitals' study. Psychological Medicine 11, 765–782.

Jelinkova, A. (1988). Coping with noise in noise sensitive subjects. Noise 88: Noise as a Public Health Problem. Vol. 3: Performance, Behaviour, Animal, Combined Agents and Community Responses (ed. B. Berglund), pp. 27–30. Swedish Council for Building Research: Stockholm.

Job, R. F. S. (1988). Community response to noise: a review of factors influencing the relationship between noise exposure and reaction. Journal of the Acoustic Society of America 83, 991–1001.

Johnston, D. W. & Anastasiades, P. (1990). The relationship between heart rate and mood in real life. Journal of Psychosomatic Research 34, 21–27.

Jonah, B. A., Bradley, J. S. & Dawson, N. E. (1981). Predicting individual subjective responses to traffic noise. Journal of Applied Psychology 66, 490–501.

Jones, D. M., Chapman, A. J. & Auburn, T. C. (1981). Noise in the environment: a social perspective. Journal of Environmental Psychology 1, 43–59.

Jonnson, E. (1964). Annoyance reactions to external environmental factors in different sociological groups. Acta Sociologica 7, 229–263.

Kasl, S. V. (1984). Life stress and health. In Health Care and Human Behaviour, pp. 41–71. Academic Press: London.

Kay, D. W. K. & Roth, M. (1961). Environmental and hereditary factors in the schizophrenias of old age. Journal of Mental Science 107, 649–686.

Kayan, A. & Hood, J. D. (1984). Neuro-otological manifestations of migraine. Brain 107, 1123–1142.

Kellner, R. & Sheffield, B. F. (1973). A self-rating scale of distress. *Psychological Medicine* 3, 88–100.

Keshavan, M. S., Channabasavanna, S. M. & Reddy, G. N. N. (1981). Post-traumatic psychiatric disturbances: patterns and predictors of outcome. *British Journal of Psychiatry* 138, 157–160.

Kipper, D. A. (1977). Behaviour therapy for fears brought on by war experiences. *Journal of Consulting and Clinical Psychology* 45, 216–221.

Knipschild, P. & Oudshoorn, N. (1977). VII. Medical effects of aircraft noise: drug survey. *International Archives of Occupational and Environmental Health* 40, 97–100.

Kokokusha, D. (1973). *Report of Investigation of Living Environment around Osaka International Airport.* Aircraft Nuisance Prevention Association: Japan.

Kryter, K. D. (1970). *The Effects of Noise on Man.* Academic Press: New York.

Kryter, K. D. (1985). *The Effects of Noise on Man.* Academic Press: London.

Kryter, K. D. (1990). Aircraft noise and social factors in psychiatric hospital admission rates: a re-examination of some data. *Psychological Medicine* 20, 395–411.

Lader, M. H. & Wing, L. (1966). *Physiological Measures, Sedative Drugs, and Morbid Anxiety.* Oxford University Press: London.

Langdon, F. J. (1976a). Noise nuisance caused by road traffic in residential areas: part II. *Journal of Sound and Vibration* 47, 265–282.

Langdon, F. J. (1976b). Noise nuisance caused by road traffic in residential areas: part I. *Journal of Sound and Vibration* 47, 243–263.

Langdon, F. J. (1976c). Noise nuisance caused by road traffic in residential areas: part III. *Journal of Sound and Vibration* 49, 241–256.

Langdon, J. (1987). Some residual problems in noise nuisance: a brief review. In *Developments in Toxicology and Environmental Science* (ed. H. S. Koelega), pp. 321–329. Elsevier: Amsterdam.

Langdon, F. J., Buller, I. B. & Scholes, W. E. (1981). Noise from neighbours and the sound insulation of party walls in houses. *Journal of Sound and Vibration* 79, 205–228.

Loeb, M. (1986). *Noise and Human Efficiency.* Wiley: Chichester.

Lynn, R. (1966). *Attention, Arousal and the Orientation Reaction.* Pergamon: Oxford.

McKennell, A. C. (1963). *Aircraft Noise Annoyance Around London (Heathrow) Airport.* Central Office of Information S.S. 337: London.

McKennell, A. C. (1977). *Community Response to Concorde Flights Round London (Heathrow) Airport.* Social and Community Planning Research: London.

McLean, E. K. & Tarnopolsky, A. (1977). Noise, discomfort and mental health. *Psychological Medicine* 7, 19–62.

McNally, R. J. (1987). Preparedness and phobias: a review. *Psychological Bulletin* 101, 283–303.

Mahapatra, S. B. (1974). Psychiatric and psychosomatic illness in the deaf. *British Journal of Psychiatry* 125, 450–451.

Meecham, W. C. & Shaw, N. (1979). Effects of jet noise on mortality rates. *British Journal of Audiology* 13, 77–80.

Meecham, W. C. & Smith, H. G. (1977). Effects of jet aircraft noise on mental hospital admissions. *British Journal of Audiology* 11, 81–85.

Meijer, H., Knipschild, P. & Salle, M. (1985). Road traffic noise annoyance in Amsterdam. *International Archives of Occupational and Environmental Health* 56, 285–297.

Melamed, S., Najenson, T., Luz, T., Jucha, E. & Green, M. (1988). Noise annoyance, industrial noise exposure and psychological stress symptoms among male and female workers. *Noise 88: Noise as a Public Health Problem. Vol. 2: Hearing, Communication, Sleep and Non-auditory Physiological Effects* (ed. B. Berglund), pp. 315–320. Swedish Council for Building Research: Stockholm.

Mischel, W. (1968). *Personality and Assessment.* Wiley: Chichester.

Moehler, U. (1988). Community response to railway noise: a review of social surveys. *Journal of Sound and Vibration* 120, 321–332.

Moran, S. L. V., Gunn, W. J. & Loeb, M. (1981). Annoyance by aircraft noise and fear of overflying aircraft in relation to attitudes toward the environment and community. *Journal of Auditory Research* 21, 217–225.

Moreira, N. M. & Bryan, M. E. (1972). Noise annoyance susceptibility. *Journal of Sound and Vibration* 21, 449–462.

Morrow, G. R. & Labrum, A. N. (1978). The relationship between psychological and physiological measures of anxiety. *Psychological Medicine* 8, 95–101.

Najenson, T., Melamed, S., Korn, C., Jucha, A. & Green, M. (1988). Auditory and non-auditory effects of industrial noise. *Noise 88. Noise as a Public Health Problem, Vol. 2. Hearing, Communication, Sleep and Non-auditory Physiological Effects* (ed. B. Berglund), pp. 325–335. Swedish Council for Building Research: Stockholm.

Nyström, S. & Lindegård, B. (1975). Depression: predisposing factors. *Acta Psychiatrica Scandinavica* 51, 77–87.

Öhman, A., Eriksson, A., Fredriksson, M., Hugdahl, K. & Olofsson, C. (1974). Habituation of the electrodermal orienting reaction to potentially phobic and supposedly neutral stimuli in normal human subjects. *Biological Psychology* 2, 85–93.

Öhman, A., Dimberg, U. & Ost, L. G. (1985). Animal and social phobias: biological constraints on learned fear responses. In *Theoretical Issues in Behaviour Therapy* (ed. S. Reiss and R. R. Bootzin), pp. 123–178. Academic Press: Orlando.

Öhrström, E. (1982). *On the Effects of Noise with Special Reference to Subjective Evaluation and Regularity.* Department of Environmental Hygiene: Göteborg, Sweden.

Öhrström, E. (1989). Sleep disturbance, psychosocial and medical symptoms – a pilot survey among persons exposed to high levels of road traffic noise. *Journal of Sound and Vibration* 133, 117–128.

Öhrström, E. & Bjorkman, M. (1988). Effect of noise-disturbed sleep – a laboratory study on habituation and subjective noise sensitivity. *Journal of Sound and Vibration* 122, 277–290.

Öhrström, E., Rylander, R. & Bjorkman, N. (1988a). Effects of night time road traffic noise – an overview of laboratory and field studies on noise dose and subjective noise sensitivity. *Journal of Sound and Vibration* 127, 441–448.

Öhrström, E., Bjorkman, M. & Rylander, R. (1988b). Noise annoyance with regard to neurophysiological sensitivity, subjective noise sensitivity and personality variables. *Psychological Medicine* 18, 605–611.

OPCS. (1971). *Second Survey of Aircraft Noise Annoyance Around London (Heathrow) Airport.* HMSO: London.

Pearson, R. G., Hart, F. D. & O'Brien, J. F. (1974). *Individual Differences in Human Annoyance Response to Noise.* Ergonomics (NASA CR-14491), North Carolina State University, Raleigh.

Philips, M. C. & Hunter, M. (1982). A laboratory technique for the assessment of pain behaviour. *Journal of Behavioral Medicine* 5, 283–294.

Poenaru, S., Rouhani, S., Poggi, D., Moch, A., Colas, C., Cohen, E., Blacker, C., Belon, J. P., Gauge, P. & Dall'Ava-Santucci, J. (1987). Study of the pathophysiological effects of chronic exposure to environmental noise in man. *Acoustic Letters* 11, 80–87.

Pulles, T., Biesiot, W. & Stewart, R. (1988). Adverse effects of environmental noise on health: an interdisciplinary approach. *Noise 88: Noise as a Public Health Problem.* (See Najenson et al. 1988).

Raps, C. S., Peterson, C., Jonas, M. & Seligman, M. E. P. (1982). Patient behaviour in hospitals: helplessness, reactance or both? *Journal of Personality and Social Psychology* 42, 1036–1041.

Raw, G. J. & Griffiths, I. D. (1988). Individual differences in response to road traffic noise. *Journal of Sound and Vibration and* 121, 463–471.

Richardson, M. W. & Kuder, G. F. (1939). The calculation of test reliability coefficient's based on the method of rational equivalence. *Journal of Educational Psychology* 30, 681–687.

Rojahn, J. & Gerhards, F. (1986). Subjective stress sensitivity and physiological responses to an aversive auditory stimulus in migraine and control subjects. *Journal of Behavioral Medicine* 9, 203–212.

Rövekamp, A. J. M. (1983). Physiological effects of environmental noise on normal and more sound-sensitive human beings. *Proceedings of the IVth International Congress on Noise as a Public*

Health Problem (ed. G. Rossi), 605–614. Centro Ricerche e Studi Amplifon: Milano.

Rushton, J. P., Jackson, D. N. & Paunonen, S. V. (1981). Personality: nomothetic or idiographic? A response to Kenrick and Stringfield. *Psychological Review* 88, 582–589.

Rylander, R., Sörenson, S. & Kajland, A. (1972). Annoyance reactions from aircraft noise exposure. *Journal of Sound and Vibration* 24, 419–444.

Schulz, T. J. (1978). Synthesis of social surveys on noise annoyance. *Journal of Acoustic Society of America* 64, 377–405.

Shepherd, M. (1974). Pollution and mental health, with particular reference to the problem of noise. *Psychiatrica Clinica* 7, 226–236.

Shigehisa, T. & Gunn, W. J. (1979). Annoyance response to recorded aircraft noise. III. In relation to personality. *Journal of Auditory Research* 19, 41–45.

Smith, A. P. & Broadbent, D. E. (1981). Noise and levels of processing. *Acta Psychologica* 47, 129.

Smith, A. P. & Stansfeld, S. A. (1986). Aircraft noise exposure, noise sensitivity and everyday errors. *Environment and Behavior* 18, 214–226.

Sokolov, E. N. (1963). *Perception and the Conditioned Reflex.* Pergamon: Oxford.

Spitzer, R. L., Endicott, J. & Robins, E. (1978). *Research Diagnostic Criteria*, 3rd edn. New York State Psychiatric Institute: New York.

Stansfeld, S. A., Clark, C. R., Jenkins, L. M. & Tarnopolsky, A. (1985a). Sensitivity to noise in a community sample. I. The measurement of psychiatric disorder and personality. *Psychological Medicine* 15, 243–254.

Stansfeld, S. A., Clark, C. R., Jenkins, L. M., Turpin, G. & Tarnopolsky, A. (1985b). Sensitivity to noise in a community sample. II. The measurement of psychophysiological indices. *Psychological Medicine* 15, 255–263.

Stansfeld, S. A. (1989). Noise sensitivity and psychiatric disorder in man: epidemiological and psychophysiological studies. Ph.D. thesis, University of London.

Stephens, S. D. G. (1970). Personality and the slope of loudness function. *Quarterly Journal of Experimental Psychology* 22, 9–13.

Stephens, S. D. G. & Powell, C. A. (1978). Laboratory and Community Studies of Aircraft Noise Effects. *Noise as a Public Health Problem* (ed. J. V. Tobias), pp. 488–494. ASHA Report 10. American Speech-Language-Hearing Association.

Syme, S. L. (1991). Control and health: a personal perspective. *Journal of Mind–Body Health* 7, 16–27.

Tarnopolsky, A. & Clark, C. (1984). Environmental noise and mental health. In *Mental Health and the Environment* (ed. H. Freeman), pp. 250–270. Churchill Livingstone: London.

Tarnopolsky, A. & Morton-Williams, J. (1980). *Aircraft Noise and Prevalence of Psychiatric Disorders, Research Report.* Social and Community Planning Research, 35 Northampton Square, London EC1.

Tarnopolsky, A., Barker, S. M., Wiggins, R. D. & McLean, E. K. (1978). The effect of aircraft noise on the mental health of a community sample: a pilot study. *Psychological Medicine* 8, 219–233.

Tarnopolsky, A., Watkins, G. & Hand, D. J. (1980). Aircraft noise and mental health. I. Prevalence of individual symptoms. *Psychological Medicine* 10, 683–698.

Taylor, S. M. (1984). A path model of aircraft noise annoyance. *Journal of Sound and Vibration* 96, 243–260.

Thomas, J. R. & Jones, D. M. (1982). Individual differences in noise annoyance and the uncomfortable loudness level. *Journal of Sound and Vibration* 82, 289–304.

Thompson, S. J. (1983). Effect of noise on the cardiovascular system: appraisal of epidemiologic evidence. In *Proceedings of the IVth International Congress, Noise as a Public Health Problem.* (ed. Rossi, G.), vol. I, pp. 711–714. Centro Ricerche e Studi Amplifon: Milano.

Thompson, S. J. (1991). Extra-aural health effects of chronic noise exposure in man. Proceedings of Noise and Disease Symposium, Berlin (unpublished manuscript).

TRACOR (1970). *Community Reaction to Airport Noise I+II (253-004).* Austin, Texas.

Turner, J. R., Girdler, S. S., Sherwood, A. & Light, K. C. (1990). Cardiovascular responses to behavioral stressors: laboratory-field generalization and inter-task consistency. *Journal of Psychosomatic Research* 34, 581–589.

Turpin, G. & Siddle, D. A. T. (1978). Cardiac and forearm plethysmographic responses to high intensity auditory stimuli. *Biological Psychology* 6, 267–282.

Turpin, G. & Siddle, D. A. T. (1983). Effects of stimulus intensity on cardiovascular activity. *Psychophysiology* 20, 611–624.

Vallet, M. & François, J. (1982). Evaluation physiologique et psychosociologique de l'effect du bruit d'avion sur le sommeil. *Travail Humain* 45, 155–168.

Vallet, M., Maurin, M., Page, M. A., Favre, B. & Pachiaudi, G. (1978). Annoyance from and habituation to road traffic noise from urban expressways. *Journal of Sound and Vibration* 60, 423–440.

Van Dijk, F. J. H. (1986). Non-auditory effects of noise in industry. II. A review of the literature. *International Archives of Occupational and Environmental Health* 58, 325–332.

Von Wright, J. & Vauras, M. (1980). Interactive effects of noise and neuroticism on recall from semantic memory. *Scandinavian Journal of Psychology* 21, 97–101.

Waddell, P. A. & Gronwall, D. M. A. (1984). Sensitivity to light and sound following minor head injury. *Acta Neurologica Scandinavica* 69, 270–276.

Watkins, G., Tarnopolsky, A. & Jenkins, L. M., (1981). Aircraft noise and mental health. II. Use of medicines and health care services. *Psychological Medicine* 11, 155–168.

Watson, D. & Clark, L. A. (1984). Negative affectivity: the disposition to experience aversive emotional states. *Psychological Bulletin* 96, 465–490.

Weinstein, N. D. (1978). Individual differences in reactions to noise: a longitudinal study in a college dormitory. *Journal of Applied Psychology* 63, 458–466.

Weinstein, N. D. (1980). Individual differences in critical tendencies and noise annoyance. *Journal of Sound and Vibration* 68, 241–248.

Weinstein, N. D. (1982). Community noise problems: evidence against adaptation. *Journal of Environmental Psychology* 2, 87–97.

Wilson, A. (chairman) (1963). *Committee on the Problem of Noise. Noise, Final Report. Cmnd 2056.* HMSO: London.

Wing, J. K. & Sturt, E. (1978). *The PSE-ID-CATEGO System supplementary manual.* MRC Social Psychiatry Unit: London.

Wing, J. K., Cooper, J. E. & Sartorius, N. (1974). *The Measurement and Classification of Psychiatric Symptoms.* Cambridge University Press: London.

Noise, noise sensitivity and psychiatric disorder: epidemiological and psychophysiological studies

The examination of the effects of noise on health is at the forefront of the investigation of the impact of environmental stressors. Environmental noise has potent effects on sleep, performance and in causing emotional reactions such as annoyance. However, the evidence that noise causes psychiatric disorder in the general population is scanty. Noise sensitivity which is a measure of attitudes to noise in general is also a predictor of annoyance responses to noise. Noise sensitivity is also associated with psychiatric disorder. This raises two questions. Are people who are sensitive to noise especially vulnerable to the effects of noise? Might noise sensitivity be an indicator of vulnerability to psychiatric disorder caused by noise?

In a 6-year follow-up study of 77 high and low noise sensitive women identified from the West London Survey around London's Heathrow airport noise sensitivity was associated with neuroticism and psychiatric disorder, was stable over time and was a powerful predictor of noise annoyance responses. It was not clear from this survey whether noise sensitivity preceded psychiatric disorder or was a consequence of psychiatric disorder. To attempt to answer this, noise sensitivity was examined in a further study of 123 depressed hospital in-patients and out-patients in relation to recovery over a 4-month period. Depressed patients became less noise sensitive as they recovered but in general they remained highly noise sensitive compared to a group of 82 age- and sex-matched non-depressed control subjects. The 'subjective' psychological measurements were complemented by 'objective' psychophysiological laboratory investigation of reactions to noise in a subsample of depressed patients. Noise sensitive people tended to have higher levels of tonic physiological arousal, more phobic and defence/startle responses and lower habituation to noise.

It is argued that noise sensitive people attend more readily to noise, perceive more threat from noise and may react more to noise than less sensitive people. Noise sensitivity appears to be a self-perceived indicator of vulnerability to stressors in general not only noise, linked to perception of environmental threat and lack of environmental control combined with a tendency to negative affectivity.

19. Community-based psychiatry: long-term patterns of care in South-Verona *edited by* **M. Tansella** (1991)

20. Schizophrenia: manifestations, incidence and course in different cultures *by* **A. Jablensky, N. Sartorius, G. Ernberg, M. Anker, A. Korten, J. E. Cooper, R. Day** and **A. Bertelsen** (1991)

21. A diagnostic analysis of the Casebooks of Ticehurst House Asylum, 1845–1890 *by* **Trevor H. Turner** (1992)

22. Noise, noise sensitivity and psychiatric disorder: epidemiological and psychophysiological studies *by* **Stephen A. Stansfeld** (1992)

Printed in the United States
By Bookmasters